PRAISE FOR THIS BOOK

"If you're looking for a miracle in your life, this book could be it. It is a must-read for anyone interested in energizing their mind, healing their body, and activating their spirit. Use it well, discover your true self, and bask in the light of Universal love. We need this book now more than ever!"

DHARMA SINGH KHALSA, MD
leading researcher and president of the Alzheimer's Research and Prevention Foundation; bestselling author of *Meditation as Medicine*

"Karena and Dharm invite us to dissolve the beliefs that keep us feeling lost using the simple magic of kundalini breathwork, so we can hear the sometimes barely-audible voice of our own intuition and follow our grace."

ELENA BROWER
author of *The Art of Attention* and *Practice You*

"*Essential Kundalini Yoga* is a book for first-timers, as well as long-time practitioners . . . The easy-to-follow explanations in this book bridge the detailed science of Western medicine with Eastern philosophies from experts in the field of health, well-being, and mindset."

PAUL J. GILSON, MD
clinical professor of neurology, Robert Woods Johnson School of Medicine

"Karena Virginia and Dharm Khalsa illuminate a complex and rich practice with friendliness, joy, and love, all while staying true to the heart of the kundalini yoga tradition. This book gives practitioners of all levels the skills and confidence they need for a powerful and nurturing kundalini yoga practice."

SEANE CORN
internationally celebrated yoga teacher, social activist, and cofounder of Off the Mat, Into the World

"Conventional medicine's tools cannot meet the complexity of the modern condition, so we are reaching for ancient technology. As a holistic physician, I enthusiastically recommend these practices to my patients and have been nothing short of amazed at the results. *Essential Kundalini Yoga* is an urgently needed guide to self-initiation and healing in today's world."

KELLY BROGAN, MD
New York Times bestselling author of *A Mind of Your Own*

"Karena Virginia and Dharm Khalsa have written a beautiful book of timeless wisdom that brings the magic of kundalini yoga as taught by Yogi Bhajan to a new audience. As a teacher and devotee of this practice and its transformational power for many years, I am delighted that this book has been brought forth as a gift of love for new yogis to discover and to become inspired within its practice."

KRISTEN EYKEL, CHT
TV personality and author of *Planning for Success*

"This book is an intelligent insight into the miracles and healing of kundalini yoga that will inspire not only the beginner, but the regular practitioner as well."

SNATAM KAUR
musician and author of *Original Light*

"Karena and Dharm have created a gem here in this book. It demonstrates how kundalini yoga can be used to connect the higher frequencies, the ocean of love, and your abilities of attraction. I highly recommend it for those who are called to break through limiting beliefs and enter the world of all possibilities."

GURU SINGH
internationally recognized master spiritual teacher and musician; author of *Buried Treasures*

"*Essential Kundalini Yoga* encapsulates a rare, modern-mind translation of ancient technology, ripe with palatable, bite-sized nuggets of wisdom . . . First-time students to seasoned practitioners will get that instant sense of calm and inspiration, regardless of which page they flip to or how much time is spent indulging in any given sitting."

JAMIE LEE
TV and radio host, KRI-certified educator, and healthy lifestyle expert

"Karena and Dharm have created a masterpiece that enables us to move beyond the limitations of the mind so we can live in our brilliance and share our light with the world . . . *Essential Kundalini Yoga* is a simple guidebook to help you blossom into your full form instead of settling for a mediocre life or hiding behind humility. This book reveals simple tips for the modern world which were kept secret in the Holy Land of India for thousands of years. It is a treasure to have and to share."

RESHMA THAKKAR
featured on Oprah Winfrey's *Belief* television event and founder of Made with a Purpose

"There are very many books out there that tell you what to do, but very few crafted as well as this that explain and demonstrate how to work with these esoteric techniques. The how-to instructions for the postures, breath, and visualization in each pose allows deep access to the experiential aspect of our Divine Nature and its connection to the Divine Sacred. My experience with this book was that of being gently guided to the inner door, being handed the magic keys, and finding inside the crown jewels of the ancient and sacred arts and sciences."

J. MICHAEL WOOD
certified master of Medical Qigong

"A beautifully presented book, written with sensitivity both to yogic principles and practice and to the need of our times to undertake what we do with an attitude of loving kindness and a gentle nurturing of self.

The authors have provided . . . an easily accessible kundalini regime for novices to adopt. While adhering to their expert knowledge of this discipline, they have produced this delightful book as a testament to the best yogic traditions made simple. I highly recommend this book for anyone who is drawn to yoga, be they newbies or more seasoned proponents.

There are gems embedded herein which belie the simplicity of the content."

NICKY HAMID, PhD
author of *All You Can Be* and "professor of happiness"

"Everyone can benefit from practicing kundalini yoga. This book will show you the way to unlock strengths you never knew you had."

PARVATI SHALLOW
winner of CBS's hit show *Survivor*

"Kundalini yoga has given me the tools to thrive in my life. I am thrilled to see a book written about kundalini yoga that is for everyone. The technology of kundalini yoga has the ability to uplift and inspire all of us. I believe that this book will give you tools to elevate your life."

CARRIE-ANNE MOSS
actor, Trinity in the *Matrix* series; founder of Annapurna Living and the Fierce Grace Collective

"A beautifully presented, simply written, and accessible portrait of kundalini yoga from the authors' unique perspective."

ALAN ARKIN
Academy Award®-winning actor and bestselling author of *An Improvised Life*

ESSENTIAL
KUNDALINI
YOGA

ESSENTIAL KUNDALINI YOGA

AN INVITATION TO RADIANT HEALTH,
UNCONDITIONAL LOVE, AND THE AWAKENING
OF YOUR ENERGETIC POTENTIAL

KARENA VIRGINIA & DHARM KHALSA

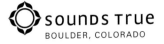
BOULDER, COLORADO

Sounds True, Inc.
Boulder, CO 80306

Published 2017

Cover and book design by Rachael Murray
Cover and interior photos © Brooks Freehill

Printed in Canada

Names: Virginia, Karena, author. | Khalsa, Dharm, 1959- author.
Title: Essential kundalini yoga : an invitation to radiant health,
      unconditional love, and the awakening of your energetic potential /
      Karena Virginia and Dharm Khalsa.
Description: Boulder, CO : Sounds True, Inc., [2017]
Identifiers: LCCN 2016021344 (print) | LCCN 2016031630 (ebook) |
      ISBN 9781622036622 (pbk.) | ISBN 9781622037308 (ebook)
Subjects: LCSH: Kuònòdalinåi. | Spiritual life.
Classification: LCC BL1238.56.K86 V57 2017 (print) | LCC BL1238.56.K86
      (ebook) | DDC 204/.36—dc23
LC record available at https://lccn.loc.gov/2016021344

10 9 8 7 6 5 4 3 2 1

WE DEDICATE THIS BOOK TO Karena's father, Giulio Ferrari, and Dharm's mother, Osa Skotting Maclane. Giulio was Karena's first spiritual teacher. He taught her to love with all the love in her heart and showed her the everyday beauty of giving to the Divine by giving to others. His spirit was tangible as we opened our hearts and poured our love into the delicate balance of words. Osa was Dharm's first yoga teacher. She passed on into the light as this book was being created, and her sense of aesthetic balance, patience, and grace runs deeply through the pages. She lived her life as an artist creating from her heart to her hands.

Both Giulio and Osa would have loved to have seen the finished book and hold it in their hands. Their memory reminds us every day that compassion, kindness, and generosity are essential ingredients for a fulfilled life.

We also dedicate this book to our amazing spouses, Charles Virginia and Gurukirn Khalsa, for their support and inspiration, which made this book possible. Your unwavering love is reflected in these words. To our children, Gabriella and Christian Virginia, and Hari Rai and Sahib Simran Khalsa, who are the joy in our hearts dancing out into the world. We love you to the moon and back for infinity, and you will always be our babies and our teachers at the same time.

To Mommy, Dad, Stephi, Robert, William, and Gitte. We love you forever. To all those who share our hearts and connect with us in one beautiful tapestry.

To Yogi Bhajan for openly sharing these sacred teachings, and encouraging us to dwell within the stream of grace that comes from timeless truth. We dedicate this book to you, the entire Golden Chain of teachers, and to your transformative prescence in our lives. We are forever grateful.

To the millions of angels who dance and sing around our globe reminding us that we are all so very similar, and we are all so very loved. Always.

We would like to make an extra special dedication to Karena's nephew, Michael James Ferrari, who passed on into the arms of the infinite during the time of writing this book. His sweet smile and loving heart will always be remembered, and he lives within many of the words in this book. We pray that his soul touches and heals the lives of teenagers, and that we may be conduits helping many others find their way.

Finally, with all the love in our hearts, we dedicate this book to you, dear reader, for holding these words close to your heart. We pray it touches your life and inspires you to touch another. May you be blessed with love forever.

CONTENTS

INTRODUCTION

EACH OF US HAS AMAZING potential for creating health, happiness, love, and a life of fulfillment. Deep in our hearts, we know we have the ability to activate and generate a life of our highest calling. The question is: Are we allowing the magnificent brightness of our true selves to shine, or are we hiding the radiance we were born with? Just as a diamond needs light to sparkle, our own true self needs the release of its inner light to be fulfilled.

This book is about clearing our energetic restrictions so our true selves shine as wonderfully as they can, in accord with our natural, inherent ability. The ancient practices of kundalini yoga are incredibly effective tools in this modern age for activating the elusive, hidden release of magnetism we are born with. The exercises open up energy pathways within our body, so we can experience vibrant health, abundance, love, empathy, intuition, and an expanded sense of connection with others.

Many people are experiencing a tangible soul-level drive for self-actualization. It feels like a voice deeply connected with the center of our being that is waiting to be heard. But although we feel it calling inside, we suppress it with self-limiting beliefs, and our unique brilliance remains hidden beneath layers of politeness and emotional armor. We may distract ourselves with our busy lives, stifle our yearnings, and go to sleep feeling so unfulfilled night after night that we become used to it. There are a hundred ways to hide the sensitive, beautiful nature of who we are.

In this era, many of us are noticing an inner voice persistently reminding us to leave behind our fears and step into the magnificence that we naturally possess. And the urging, calling, and whispering of this inner voice can no longer be ignored. If you have picked up this book, chances are that you are hearing it yourself.

THE SECRET YOGA OF ENERGY

Kundalini yoga is an ancient, time-tested system of exercise and meditation that boosts our energy, synchronizes the impulses of our nervous system, releases energetic blockages, balances our hormones, and uplifts our attitude to allow the pure radiance of our authentic self to shine. While other branches of yoga focus primarily on physical postures, kundalini yoga focuses on how the postures alter our energy and mind-set. Postures, movement, breathing, meditation, mantras, and lifestyle come together to bring about remarkable transformations of personal energy. The term *kundalini* refers to the concentrated living energy that opens up our potential. It is an energy that is dormant yet calls us to be awakened within. Once activated, it permeates us, energizes our cells to bring health and vitality, and connects our consciousness with the infinite. The techniques of kundalini yoga were developed over the course of thousands of years and are highly effective tools for opening up our energy pathways so the right amount of energy at the right frequency can flow smoothly through our entire being.

Kundalini yoga works on the principle that our physical body and our energy move hand in hand. What we do with our body has a parallel effect on our energy, and, likewise, what we do with our energy has a parallel effect on our body. For example, tightness in our hamstrings is actually a blockage in the energy that otherwise would be flowing through that area of our body. We call that tightness an *opacity* because it is blocking the flow of inner light. Using the ancient techniques of kundalini yoga to stretch the muscle or move a limb through the energy field that surrounds our body, we can release the corresponding blocked-up energy. Our inner light can then start flowing into an area where it was restricted before. The resulting effect on our body and mind is absolutely profound. Not only does the muscle itself become more limber, but our consciousness shifts, our mind becomes clearer, and the new energy optimizes our functioning at the genetic level. As the light flows through our energy field, our awareness comes alive. Our energy level soars, and, like a flower emerging from the soil after a long, cold winter, we feel alive and hopeful.

Kundalini yoga was kept secret in India for thousands of years, taught only to devotees who were deemed worthy. In the 1960s, Yogi Bhajan moved from his home country of India to the United States. He began teaching kundalini yoga as a technology for self-improvement, and it quickly became popular. He authored more than thirty books and traveled extensively, teaching kundalini yoga around the globe until his passing in 2004. The authors have studied kundalini yoga extensively. In this book, for historical accuracy, we have sourced the exercises so you can see whether an exercise was taught by Yogi Bhajan, is a classic from the ages, or is a visualization we bring to help explain a topic.

THE KUNDALINI SPIRIT

Practicing kundalini yoga often results in a natural sensation of oneness with a universal force greater than our limited sense of self. Yet kundalini yoga is not a religion, can be practiced by anyone with any spiritual belief, and does not require any particular spiritual philosophy. It is typical for the practices to enhance one's feelings of spirituality, whether you belong to a formal religion or not. Flashes of insight, cosmic breakthroughs, tears of joy, and sobs of surrender are normal occurrences when the wondrous flood of our own energy is finally allowed to emerge through the layers of shielding we have put up all our lives. We encourage you to allow yourself to be swept up in the gift of spiritual experience rather than resisting out of fear. In fact, it is high time to give up the fear of your own brightness. Throughout this book, we use the terms God, *the infinite*, *spirit source*,

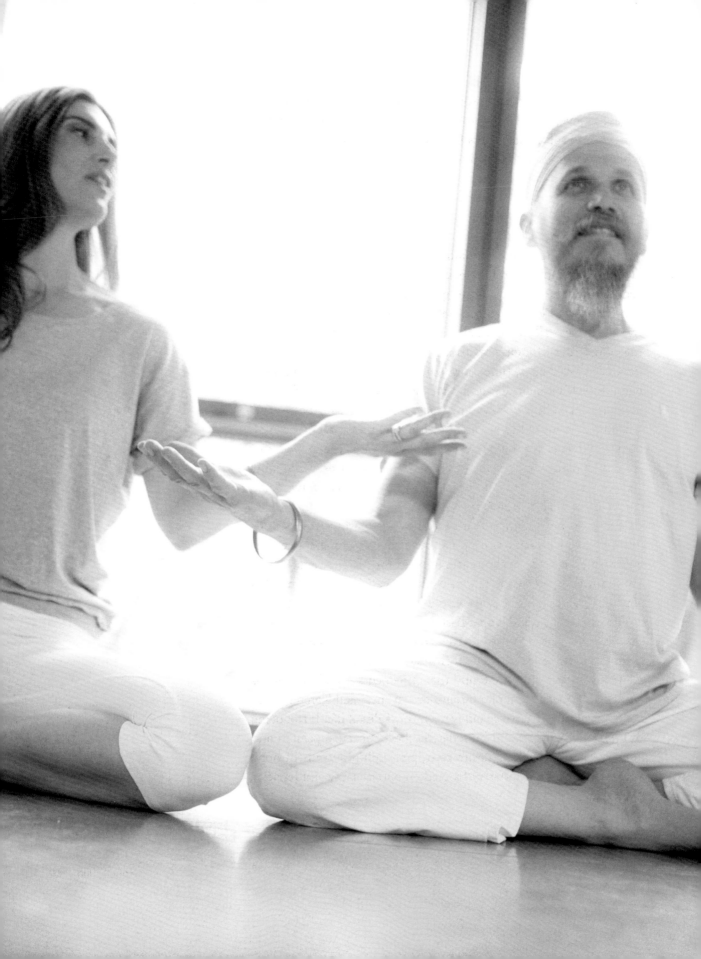

and *the universe* to reflect the oneness of universal spirit in kundalini yoga. However, these are simply terms, and you are invited to carry the sense of spirit that works for you from this book into your life while leaving the rest behind.

WHO WE ARE

We have been practicing kundalini yoga for a combined total of fifty years. In our teaching and travels, we have found people everywhere yearning for the same thing: to give love and receive love with a depth and abundance that reaches their soul. Love is the common thread through all hearts in all cultures. Yet many feel caught in a life of perpetual longing, as though something were missing. We have been asked many times how to use kundalini yoga as a means to end the cycle of emptiness and yearning many people feel. We have also been asked how to eliminate fear and insecurity so one can find a way to align his or her life with health, happiness, and peace. This book aims to answer these questions—to show you the miracle that is waiting to blossom in your life and how the practices of kundalini yoga can help you allow it to unfold. For it is in the allowing of new energy flows that we transform.

While she had practiced hatha yoga since she was a teen, Karena did not discover kundalini yoga until she was in her twenties. Working as an actor in the bustle of New York City, she found herself yearning for the soft, innocent, and angelic forces she had felt connected with as a child. When she came upon kundalini yoga in the basement of a small Upper East Side gym, she immediately knew she had come home to a practice that her soul had been searching for. She began sharing the techniques of kundalini yoga during television shoots, and she found that it helped her and her friends attract jobs, partners, and contentment. It mystified Karena to see how the practice opened so many to the miracles of life. Introducing concepts of the kundalini lifestyle to others became a passion and fulfilled Karena's lifelong desire to inspire, uplift, and instill hope in others. Within an industry focused on outer beauty and tenacity, kundalini yoga became the primary resource that helped Karena stay internally balanced and connected to the divine. Karena has always had an extremely sensitive constitution, and she credits the gift of kundalini yoga with empowering her to live through her heart with innocence and compassion. It has also enabled her to recognize that those who feel deeply are not flawed but, rather, are blessings in our world who often help others heal with the power of love and grace.

Dharm started to practice hatha yoga when he was eight years old, learning the poses from his mother. He was introduced to kundalini yoga in college and found the practices were the first that genuinely supported his intuition and feelings of universal consciousness. He soon began adding kundalini yoga to the yoga classes he taught. When he was twenty-three he sought out the master of kundalini yoga, Yogi Bhajan, as a spiritual guide. Yogi Bhajan gave him the position of *sevadar*, which is a very humble assistant on his personal staff. Dharm spent the next twenty-two years studying with him, until Yogi Bhajan's passing in 2004. In the midst of this journey, Dharm was called to the all-inclusive spirit, discipline, and loving meditative awareness of the Sikh faith, and he began wearing the traditional Sikh turban and unshorn hair. In the decade since the passing of Yogi Bhajan, Dharm has continued his devotion in alignment with Yogi Bhajan's energy as a member of the Board of Trustees of the Siri Singh Sahib Corporation, the oversight body created by Yogi Bhajan for the kundalini yoga community, and as a member of the board of directors of 3HO Foundation, the nonprofit entity that Yogi Bhajan founded in the 1960s.

ABOUT THE BOOK

This book is intended for everyone. We present the concepts and exercises in simple language that allows you to start practicing, and experiencing the power and effectiveness of the techniques, right away. We would like to demystify what can sometimes be perceived as complex. At the same time, we offer a depth of information that dives below the surface and into the basis behind the exercises. If you already have experience with kundalini yoga, you may find a fresh approach as we immerse ourselves in the deep, soul-level energy that is at the core of the exercises and meditations.

Quantum physicists have found that energy is the essence of all there is. We wrote *Essential Kundalini Yoga* to make the concepts of awakening our personal energy understandable and accessible to everyone. Kundalini yoga does not have to be mysterious. It is an ancient tradition with practices that could fill thousands of pages and a lifetime of study, but we have selected techniques that we have found to be especially effective at moving personal energy and optimizing health and consciousness in a way that helps you step into your potential. We share techniques learned from Yogi Bhajan that we have found to be most powerful in our own practices. We have included exercises and visualizations from our own experiences to help you connect with your energy field. For many of the practices, we have suggested modifications that offer the benefits of the technique in a less strenuous position.

This book is organized into three parts. Part 1 is about your personal bioenergy and how it interacts with your nerves, hormones, and brain chemistry. You will learn about the energy pathways in your body and about how your personal energy creates a vibration that flows into the space around your body—your electromagnetic field—impacting the physical world surrounding you. We will share special breathing techniques and will explain how to use sound to release blocked pathways and change your vibration in profound and healing ways.

In part 2 we dive into the depth of the practice, first with yoga basics and then plunging more deeply into the beautiful embrace of energy work with classic kundalini yoga sets. This is a section you can come back to again and again. We have specifically selected exercises that allow you to uncover and activate the full power of your own magnificent self.

In part 3 we deepen into the experience of moving past inner energy blocks, opening up to the possibilities that are natural yet immensely powerful, and allowing our vibration to attract love, health, peace, and vitality. You will find many topics, from beauty secrets to a technique for overcoming sadness, all addressed from an energetic understanding.

In the final chapter, we discuss how to bring light into your daily life in a way that aligns with your distinct vibration—the unique frequency of your true self. All the practice in the world won't help unless we bring it into our lives with love and compassion and share our graciousness with one another.

YOU ARE INVITED

And the day came when the risk to remain tight in a bud
was more painful than the risk it took to blossom.
ANAÏS NIN

We all have a choice: to access the core of light that our soul has been yearning to express, opening our inner passages to allow our luminescence fully into our life, or to hide our unique way of shining behind a facade of social acceptance that we often have spent many years building. When we make the choice to uncover our true self, kundalini yoga provides exceptional tools to help us. If we practice with courage, vulnerability, and dedication, we are able to entertain a calm, centered power far beyond the ordinary.

We are inviting you to follow the path of least resistance—the path of flow. By removing energetic blocks and aligning our personal authenticity with the grace of the universe, we take the first step on the path of miracles. We invite you to begin your journey into the light of your own being.

PART 1
AN ENERGIZED BODY

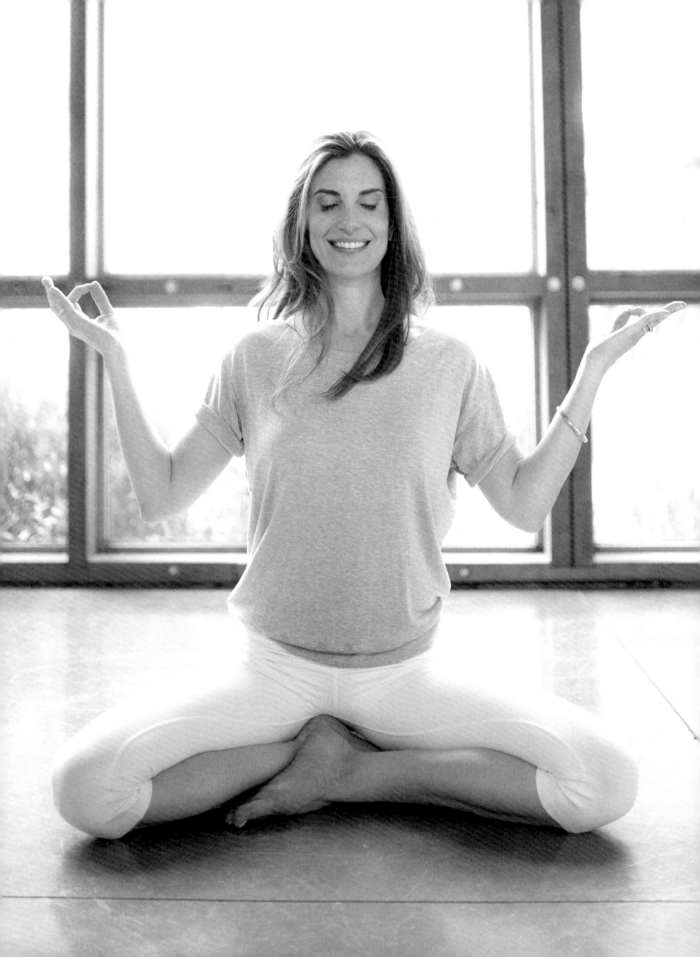

1 LET'S BE REAL

Accept yourself as you. Live within yourself so that the without can relate to you. Out of you can spring beautiful thoughts. Out of you can spring beautiful radiance. Out of you can come peace. Out of you can come God. But before anything can come out of you, it must be there. . . . Reality is living with yourself, accepting yourself, and being within yourself. That is the secret of prosperity.
YOGI BHAJAN

WE HAVE FOUND A TECHNOLOGY that has assisted us in our lives. We are not saying that life is always a rose garden, with rainbows and unicorns showing up to free us from disappointments. We are not preaching or hypothesizing a religion. We are simply sharing a technique that we have seen change people's lives.

We have witnessed miracles. We have observed people heal from life-threatening diseases. We have watched babies come into this world from parents who were told they would never conceive a child. We have seen people struggling with marriage, family, and loneliness who turned their lives around by using the techniques we are sharing in this book. We do not pretend to have all the answers to this thing called life. However, we know from our own personal experiences that this technology has worked in ways that modern science is only recently beginning to understand.

You cannot think yourself out of thinking. You cannot think yourself out of obsessing. You cannot think yourself out of fear. But you can change your energy to change your thoughts. Changing our energy to change our lives is the concept behind this book.

Through our investigation of the astonishing miracles we have observed, we are convinced that the energy field in and around the physical body and the breath are the missing links in the world of wellness. The ideas in this book may be new to you, but they are based on ancient practices. We invite you to step outside of old thought patterns and into the realm of possibility.

THE VIBRATION OF PRANA

Prana is the energy that flows through us to keep us alive, activating our life and giving us the ability to shine. Prana has a magnetic quality about it, a charisma of its own. When prana flows through our body with ease and without blockages, we can be radiantly healthy and unlock our fullest potential. In many ways our prana is who we are. If we could take a picture of our energy, it would be a luminous three-dimensional mandala of vibrating frequencies and harmonies reverberating through our body and through the electromagnetic field that surrounds us.

Our breath is the main delivery service that brings pranic energy to every cell and into the electromagnetic field that surrounds our body. We also have the ability to give and receive prana from other people, animals, and plants through touch, prayer, and all our interactions. Even a hug creates an exchange of prana. We gain prana from our food and even absorb it through our skin. When we fall in love and are thinking about our beloved, and as they think of us in turn, we exchange pranic energy in one of the most beautiful ways there is.

Kundalini is the concentrated form of prana of the human being. It is the power of the divine inside the human. Kundalini lies dormant at the base of the spine until the frequency required for activation is reached and blocks in our energy channels are cleared, at which point it rises through the central channel of the spine to activate our life-force. When kundalini energy is awakened, it initiates a remarkable series of events in the mind and body. The awakening integrates the energy of the soul into the physical reality of life. It sounds like a mystical process, but it is simply a matter of developing the potential for who you truly are. And we will make it as simple and straightforward as possible.

Surrounding our body is a field of energy that resonates with the bioactivity happening inside of us. Called the *electromagnetic field* or the *aura*—terms we will use interchangeably throughout the book—this field is where transformation starts. In order to change our cellular expression to one of health, the practices of kundalini yoga use prana to make the energy shifts in our magnetic field.

In this new age there is so much talk about how thoughts create our reality. This is true; however, it is prana that powers our thoughts. The mind will not shift out of stuck patterns of fear simply by thinking its way out. What we think we set in motion through the power of our prana. We shift our thoughts with our prana because our thoughts are actually energetic wave forms. It is our prana that strengthens, energizes, heals, expands, and purifies the electromagnetic field, bringing brilliance and power to it.

FOUR QUALITIES OF PRANA

When you understand who and what you are, your radiance projects into the universal radiance, and everything around you becomes creative and full of opportunity.
YOGI BHAJAN

The following four qualities of prana provide a framework for working with kundalini energy.

THE DRIVE TO ACTIVATION

We all have a calling that is compelling us to move forward on our life journey. That calling is built into prana, encouraging us to evolve. The universe wants us to awaken, and it will work with us in infinite detail toward becoming the most healthy, radiant beings that we can be. In fact, all sorts of circumstances and synchronicities transpire to assist in our awakening once we set prana in motion.

At a soul level we feel the calling and trust this support; however, we often hold ourselves back. We subconsciously fear we will re-create mistakes from our past or might not be accepted by others, so we freeze where we are and create an energetic block to our activation. Those energetic blocks become habitual, and seem daunting. But they can be dissolved by shifting the flow and vibration of our prana. Once the inner blocks are gone, the light of our true selves can shine out from the center of our being, into our body, and into the world around us. This is your personal glow that prana has the potential to activate. It is felt as our drive for self-actualization, as our soul yearns to fulfill its purpose.

FREQUENCY

Everything vibrates at a subtle frequency. The higher your frequency is, the higher your magnetism will be. The frequency of our prana is the key to our health, awareness, and attraction force. Within each of us is an energy mix of happiness and sorrows, joys and struggles, wishes and desires; we are a vibrating, three-dimensional mandala of our unique self. We are broadcasting our energy out to the world all the time.

Our mood is how we experience the vibration of our prana. Our prana always conveys a character portrait, and we can learn to shift its frequency to one of health and attraction. The seemingly magical vibration that opens our consciousness, activates our health, and awakens our potential is love. It opens shutters that otherwise remain closed, so that the light of our soul can illuminate the brilliant diamond of our being. Shifting our frequency is not always easy. We get stuck in habitual mood patterns. But through kundalini yoga practices, we can change the vibrational frequency of our energy back to its source—back to love. A cascade of remarkable benefits—emotional, physical, and spiritual—then flows forth.

RESONANCE

The scientific phenomenon of *sympathetic resonance* is a powerful secret to opening up a life that is aligned with your true self. Simply put, our inner frequency projects beyond our physical body into the electromagnetic field around us. Our *resonance* amplifies and harmonizes with similar frequencies in the world. If your electromagnetic field is vibrating with the energy of gratitude, for example, that vibration will resonate with similar frequencies in every place that is affected by your electromagnetic field, whether inside your body or in the physical environment around you. This is how our thoughts create the reality of our lives. Our thoughts create a vibration that resonates with and activates the same character it is giving out. That is why the work of shifting out of habitual unhealthy thought patterns is so essential. That work is one of the strengths of kundalini yoga.

Your own true shine and your own inspirations can serve you amazingly well if they are directed, as they attract more of the same frequency into your life. Like attracts like.

RADIANCE

Radiance is our sparkle and shine. It is the illumination emitted by our energy frequencies and is powered by prana. Our radiance vibrates through the aura and connects us to the infinite. When our radiance is healthy, we become magnetic beings who draw opportunities and success with synchronicity rather than with effort. The energy of our radiant body starts with the spin of atoms within our cells and echoes into the ends of the universe. By aligning that atomic spin with our soul's purpose, and at the same time removing the blocks and fears that restrict our energy flow, we can connect with the highest potential of our life and attract love, harmony, and grace. All of our energy has the potential for radiance.

○ GOLDEN LIGHT BREATH FOR ACTIVATING PRANA

Golden Light Breath connects us with the dynamic and magnetic flow of life energy. In the instructions below, we suggest lying on your back, but you can tune in to your prana with this breathing technique almost anywhere—while sitting at your desk, as you are walking, or when sitting still in meditation. This is a wonderful practice to do while lying down in bed before falling asleep.

1   Lie on your back and place your hands on your lower belly. As you inhale and exhale, visualize your breath as a golden light rather than invisible air.

2   Inhale and let your abdomen expand like a balloon. Slow your breath down, breathing as deeply and slowly as possible while observing the expansion of your belly. Feel that your breath is made of golden light. Fully fill every portion of your lungs on the inhale.

3   Hold your breath and let the golden light circulate through your entire body and into the field beyond your skin, around your body.

4   As you exhale, allow your belly to deflate all the way down so your belly button draws in toward your spine. Feel the golden light extending past your skin and into the space around your body and blending with all the light of the universe.

5   Hold your breath out for a few moments before slowly and consciously inhaling again. Continue inhaling and exhaling deeply and slowly with a gentle hold of the breath at each end, visualizing the breath as golden light.

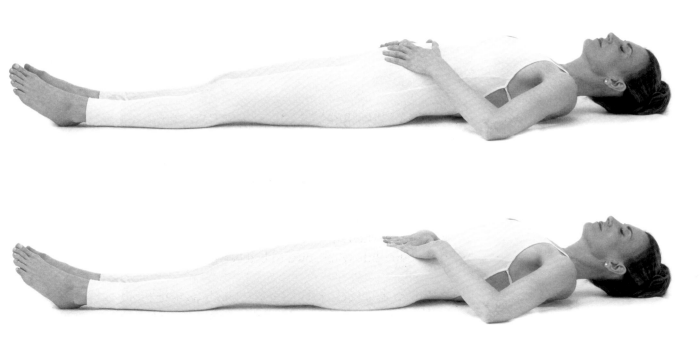

6 Feel the light entering into your being from a vast universal pool of love, flowing through your nostrils, filling your lungs, and circulating throughout your body, loving you and nourishing your cells.

7 Breathe as slowly and deeply as you can, holding your breath after each inhale and exhale, for three to eleven more minutes. Feel this light and wisdom pressing into you with every inhalation and vibrating throughout your aura as you hold your breath, loving you, nourishing you, and washing away tension. As you exhale, visualize yourself letting go of anything that is holding you back from activating your radiance.

8 To finish, observe and allow your feelings. You may have a profound positive experience after you practice this breath, or you may feel resistance and frustration. Whatever you are feeling is valuable; don't try to change it. Simply allow the sensations to arise and depart.

THE LOVE FREQUENCY PHENOMENON

Love is not a projection. Love is an attraction.
YOGI BHAJAN

More than we are a physical body, we are our energy. When our energy vibrates at the frequency of love—the energy state we are at our core—our being fills up with the most joyous, healthy vitality that we ever imagined, and our entire physiology moves into an optimized state. In the bioenvironment of love, our DNA expresses optimally in ways we never even knew could be possible. We discover new awareness and new intuition. We connect more deeply with others because we recognize that the same love that resonates in their soul resonates within ours. We find we can release an incredible amount of vibrant energy into our body and into our life. We fall in love with life, and life falls in love with us. This is the miracle.

When we vibrate at a frequency of love, our external environment shifts as well, and we become like magnets for activating our potential. When the attractive power of love fills our body and projects into our aura, it's as though what we truly desire—our true potential—seeks us out as well. This is why we coined the term *Love Frequency Phenomenon.*

Love is a human experience of the most powerful physical force of the universe. When we feel love, we are experiencing the attractive force that holds atoms together. This energetic force also brings humans together. It activates our physical body, making our cells healthy, and shines through our soul. Rather than finding it outside, we find it most accessible right inside of us. Kundalini yoga can help us tap into the love frequency phenomenon by dissolving the barriers that block our gifts from shining into the world. Love is the vibration with the power to make the impossible possible.

THE MIRACLE
SHIFTING PRANA FROM FEAR TO LOVE

When the heart gets into prayer, every beat of the heart creates a miracle.
YOGI BHAJAN

Shrinking back from who we are does not serve anyone. We may buy into the false belief that keeping our light off will allow more love to enter our lives or will somehow serve those around us. We hide so we can give others permission to shine, and then we feel hurt and disappointed when they do not give us the love we seek. We give away our light in order to please others and accept that as part of life.

There is a soul destination that cannot be put off. Sometimes it starts as an inner tickle, the soul inside teasing us to be noticed. We try to hold on to a state of numbness, but before long we find our soul asking more and more to be acknowledged, encouraged, and released.

If you have picked up this book, chances are you have felt that tickle. We have a remarkable potential to shine. The world needs each of our lights. We know it. Now is the time to start to step into our radiance.

When the light of your own soul's magnificence expands outward, resistances melt away and life begins to flow. Synchronicities happen. A wisdom is waiting to unfold that will not hurt anyone. This is your natural and most powerful state of being. Hiding your light is not.

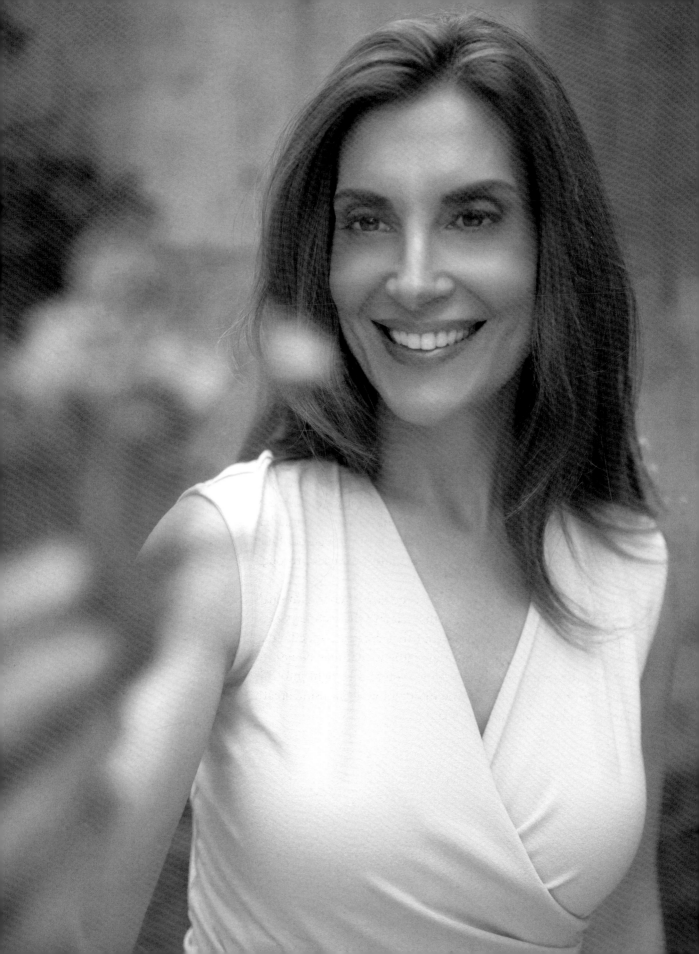

2 ENERGY BODIES

It's pleasing to discover that it isn't necessary to drive oneself forward; instead, one can simply allow oneself to move forward as blocks are removed. Thus, one becomes attracted by the future rather than propelled by the past.
DAVID HAWKINS

IN THE KUNDALINI YOGA TRADITION, the physical body is only a portion of who we are. Just as our physical body has a structure with limbs, organs, and cells, our energy has aspects that we conceive of as structural. We each have eight *chakras*, or energy centers, that resonate with the frequencies of energy that flow through our body as well as a network of energy channels, called the *nadis*, through which our prana flows.

The techniques in this chapter open the flow of energy through our chakras and nadis. You will find that a few of the techniques use a repeating *mantra*, a repetitive sound that creates a specific outcome. Others use powerful breathing methods that may be new to you. We have made it simple enough for you to dive right into this chapter, but if you would like more information about using breath and mantras please see chapters 4 and 5.

THE CHAKRAS

All light is vibration. Visible light can be separated into distinct colors by generating a rainbow. The light appears to be separate colors as its frequency changes, but blended together the frequencies form one white light. Similarly, our chakras—each a different frequency and color—express the entire spectrum of frequencies that comprise the energy of the physical body. The word *chakra* (pronounced "*chak*-rah") means "wheel" or "circle," named so by the ancient yogis to depict a wheel-shaped vibration of pranic energy.

A chakra is pure and continuous energy. It is our prana in motion, a wavelength of vibration in our electromagnetic field that contains our values, feelings, thoughts, and childhood imprints. As each of the eight chakras become energized, the physical and emotional attributes corresponding to that frequency are also energized, as is our consciousness.

Much like a tuning fork that will not sound if it is held tightly, tightness in parts of our physical body can prevent our chakras from resonating. For a tuning fork to resonate, we have to release our grip, hold it delicately, and allow the vibration to flow. This is very similar to how we work with the physical body in kundalini yoga: the "tuning fork" of each chakra is anchored to the physical body, and by releasing physical tension we also release the movement of energy.

The body holds our emotions. When we have a blocked emotion, the chakra that corresponds to the part of the body holding that emotion is also blocked. When the energy starts flowing, the blocks dissolve and the emotions open. It takes deep trust to release these blockages, but it can be done by getting the prana moving.

In the following section, we describe the character of each chakra and provide exercises that will enable you to connect with its essence.

FIRST CHAKRA: EXISTENCE

The first chakra vibrates with the most fundamental aspect of our human incarnation: the energy of existence. This is the energy center connected to the material world and primal survival. Our physical body, our health, and our habits correspond to this area.

Its anatomical equivalent is at the perineum and the base of the spine. The legs and feet are also extensions of the first chakra. The color associated with the first chakra is red.

We take on form and mission with the declaration of "I am." The way we honor our very existence affects the frequency of the first chakra. When the first chakra is balanced and flowing with prana, we feel worthy of our existence and happy to be alive. It is the fertile soil from which all else arises. When our first chakra is blocked, we may not feel valued, lovable, or entitled to occupy space. An unbalanced first chakra also leads us to compare ourselves with others and resent their existence.

○ YOGA FOR THE FIRST CHAKRA CROW POSE

When we cleanse and balance the root chakra, we boost our health, strengthen our sense of security, and increase our trust in the flow of prosperity. Crow Pose brings our pranic energy to the base of the spine, the home of the first chakra and a place where we often conceal ourselves.

1   Stand with your legs three feet apart. Feel your spine rising tall from your pelvis and your weight distributed equally between both feet on the earth below you.

2   Maintaining the position of your feet, squat down with your feet flat on the ground. We invite you to press your palms together in front of your heart as if you are praying, with your elbows inside your knees and your spine as straight as possible.

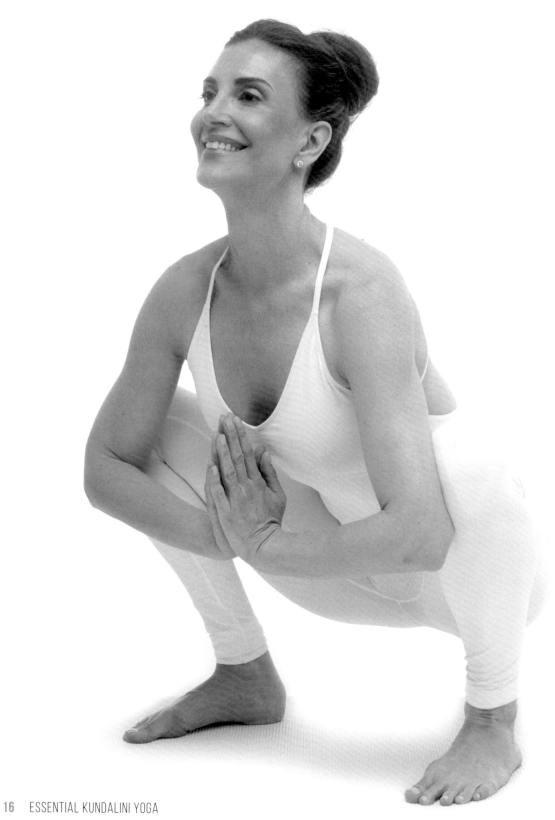

3 Inhale slowly and deeply into your abdomen, hold it for a moment, and fully empty your lungs on each exhalation. Continue holding the pose and breathing this way for thirty seconds to three minutes.

4 To finish, release the hands and bring yourself onto your back. Rest for a few minutes. Allow your breath to flow naturally again, notice the movement of prana through the physical area of the perineum and in the space surrounding your body, especially around the hips and coccyx.

SECOND CHAKRA: FEELING

The second chakra opens our incarnation into the world of trusting our sensation. We become drawn to what feels good—drawn to warmth, to touch—and in doing so become vessels of universal creativity. When we trust that what we feel is a gift from our highest consciousness, we can surrender and allow the creative force of nature to work through us. We instinctively know what to do. We trust our instincts. We go with it. We open. Conception is the first, most beautiful creativity that we are all born of. Thus, the frequency of the second chakra is represented in the physical body through the sexual and reproductive organs, the hips, and the receptive lower spine. The color associated with it is orange.

When the flow of prana through the second chakra is blocked, we no longer trust the source of our feelings. We separate our feelings from God, and our sensation becomes thought of as something negative. Many people who overly control their lives with thought have a difficult time accepting their second chakra energy because it can feel so out of control. It feels separate from their intellect because it is! The second chakra vibrates at a very deep emotional, not mental, level.

MODIFICATIONS If you have difficulty holding this position, two wonderful modifications can make it easier. First, keeping the balls of your feet on the ground, you can place a rolled-up yoga mat or blanket beneath your heels. Or, if putting your palms together causes you to fall backward, try holding on to the leg of a heavy table with both hands instead.

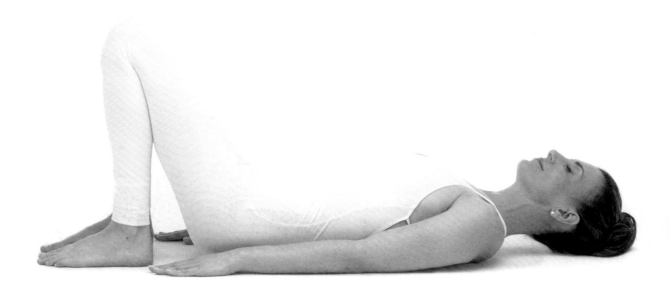

○ YOGA FOR THE SECOND CHAKRA PELVIC LIFTS

Yoga movements that open the hips and relax the pelvis encourage the flow of positive energy while releasing negative energy in the tender area of the second chakra. In this exercise we balance the energy in the lower belly by using the breath, visualization, and movement.

1 Lie down on your back with your spine flat against the ground. Feel your breath entering through your nostrils and filling your lungs; notice the rise and fall of your rib cage with each breath. Tune in to the steady, nurturing earth below you and the vastness of the sky above as you breathe.

2 Bend your knees so your soles are flat on the ground, close to your buttocks, with your knees pointing toward the sky. Place your arms alongside your torso, with the palms pressing down against the earth. Alternatively, hold on to your ankles.

3 For the first phase, inhale as you slowly raise your pelvis as high as possible, lifting your spine up off the floor one vertebra at a time, starting with the lowermost vertebrae and gradually moving up the spinal column.

4 Exhale as you slowly lower the spine back down to the starting position, feeling it reconnect, vertebra by vertebra, back down onto the ground.

5 Continue lifting up and lowering your pelvis down with a slow, steady, smooth, meditative movement. Allow your breath to lead the movement, fully filling your lungs as you inhale and stretch your spine up, fully exhaling as you lower back down. As your breath leads

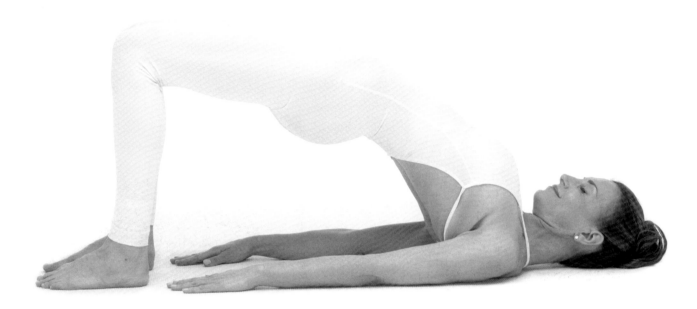

your spine, allow your spine to move the rest of your body. Visualize your breath erasing tension as you inhale and visualize your breath releasing any imbalance as you exhale. Continue for three to twenty-six lifts.

6 For the second phase, stay in the upward position while you take long, slow, and deep breaths. Completely fill the lungs and allow your rib cage to expand on each inhale. Hold your breath in for a moment after each inhalation and hold out after each exhalation. As you exhale, empty the lungs fully and allow

your rib cage to compress. Continue for three breath cycles or longer.

7 To finish, inhale deeply and hold the upward position. Imagine pent-up energy from the second chakra releasing, pouring into, and filling your lower spine; in your mind see it illuminating and infusing your entire being. Hold your inhale in and continue visualizing for as long as possible.

8 Now fully exhale while bringing your hips up a little higher. At the end of the exhale, hold the breath out for as long as you comfortably can.

9 Inhale again and slowly exhale as you lower your spine down to the floor, vertebra by vertebra, until the last parts of your body to come down are your buttocks.

10 With your back flat on the floor, turn your palms up and stretch your legs out. Stay still, taking long, slow, deep breaths, feeling the shift in your energy body, particularly around your hips, groin, and lower spine. Trust that everything you are feeling is moving through you to bring harmony in a newfound way.

THIRD CHAKRA: POWER, STABILITY, PERSEVERANCE

The navel was where we were all once connected to our mother in her womb. We completely trusted this lifeline, and every day as we grew we would draw on that connection with our mother. That sense of trust continues in our lives via the navel point. The navel point is located between the navel inward toward the base of the spine. While the navel is a physical part of our bodies, the navel point is an etheric ball of energy which holds our conscious and power as spiritual beings having a human experience. The navel point acts like a pranic reservoir, and it reverberates like sunshine radiating through our entire being. If prana is flowing easily through our third chakra, which starts just below the belly button and projects upward into the solar plexus, we have an inherent sense of being sustained energetically, giving us the power and confidence to manifest on earth. The third chakra is known in kundalini yoga as the place where true awakening happens. It is where the fire is ignited and sent to the other chakras. The color associated with this chakra is yellow.

○ YOGA FOR THE THIRD CHAKRA FRONT PLATFORM

Many people sense a pang in their stomachs when something is simply not right. We often experience our inner instinctual guidance system through feelings that seem to arise from our third chakra. There's a reason we call this a "gut reaction," and by all means it is a very important message to listen to. We can develop the sensitivity to truly listen to what the gut is expressing.

When the third chakra needs balancing, you may feel unstable in your day-to-day decisions and uncertain about your choices. The following exercise opens the flow of prana through the third chakra, balancing and sensitizing us to hear the messages we get from the solar plexus area.

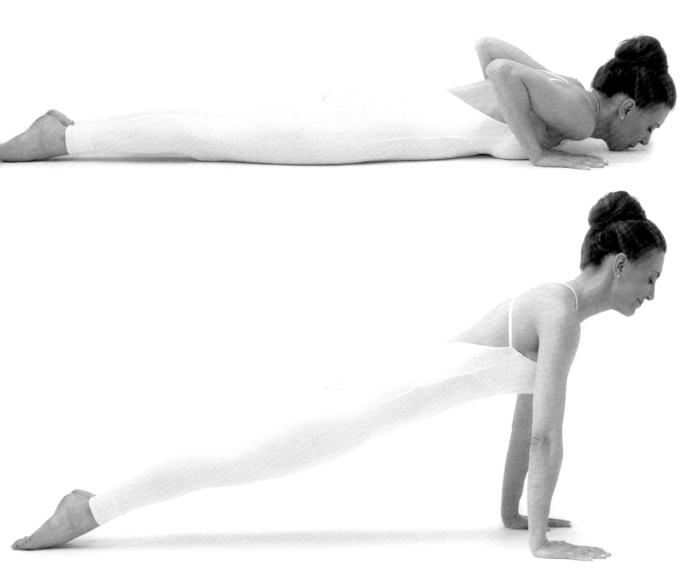

1 Lie on your stomach with your toes pointed away from your head. Bend your elbows and press your palms against the floor on either side of your body alongside your rib cage.

2 Inhale and push your body up off the floor so you are supported by your palms and the tops of your feet. Keep your heels together and the toes pointed. Look down at the floor between your hands while drawing your neck back, creating one straight line from the top of your head to your toes. Engage your abdominal muscles.

MODIFICATION If the full position is too much of a strain, keep your knees on the floor and push only your upper body up.

3 Hold the position and begin taking long, deep inhales and exhales, drawing your breath deeply into your abdomen and pushing it completely out. Imagine your breath as light. Continue for thirty seconds to three minutes, focusing on the flow of prana spiraling through your navel center.

4 To finish, bring your knees to the ground and press your glutes back toward your heels while drawing your hands alongside your hips with your palms facing upward. Rest in this Baby Pose for the same amount of time as you practiced Front Platform Pose.

FOURTH CHAKRA: LOVE

The best and most beautiful things in this world cannot be seen or even heard, but must be felt with the heart.
HELEN KELLER

The fourth chakra is the chakra of love and compassion. It corresponds to the heart, and its color is green. The heart chakra is the most powerful center in the human body. The release of kundalini energy along the short distance from the navel to the fourth chakra, or heart center, is a miracle. A huge cascade of physiological, emotional, and spiritual changes takes place when our heart is allowed to resonate with its true feelings. The heart has the capacity to transcend everything. When we pray, we pray from our heart. When memories of times with those we love make us feel sentimental, we are feeling from the heart. Our heart is our vulnerability, and we must keep it healthy with love. When we speak from our heart, we inspire others. In fact, we do not even need words to communicate from the heart. We can simply smile, and our smile expresses unity and connection.

The state of love from an activated and balanced heart center does not depend on external conditions. It becomes a self-sustaining, deep, completely natural empathy for and energetic connection with one another and with ourselves. However, when the heart chakra is imbalanced, we forget to take care of our own needs, and we may cling to others for the support we are not giving ourselves.

○ YOGA FOR THE FOURTH CHAKRA
HEART-CENTERING MEDITATION

This meditation uses a special mantra to vibrate the energy frequency of the heart center. Mantras are usually spoken or chanted out loud so that the vibration can permeate our bodies, but in this exercise you will be chanting the mantra silently, in your mind. The mantra for the Heart-Centering Meditation is an affirmation of our connectivity with all there is. The humming sound of each syllable comforts our hearts. It is pronounced "Humee Humm Brahmm Humm," and it means, "I am I, and I am divine." This mantra reminds our souls that we are part of a much greater whole and that we are loved in more ways than the mind can comprehend.

Humee
Humm
Brahmm
Humm

1   Sit on your heels in a kneeling position, keeping your spine straight. Spend a few moments feeling the flow of breath entering deeply into your lungs.

2   With your elbows extended to the sides, like wings, and forearms parallel to the ground, turn your palms toward the ground and touch your middle fingers together in front of your heart. Keep your fingers straight. Please see photo on the next page.

3   Lower your eyelids until they are almost closed and focus your gaze on the tip of your nose. This eye position is often used in kundalini yoga to focus and quiet the mind as well as activate the pituitary and pineal glands.

4   Like when you have a song in your head, listen to your inner voice silently vibrating with the mantra "Humee Hum Brahm Hum" (pronounced "hummee humm *brumm* humm"). Listen to yourself chanting as though you were moving your mouth, but without speaking or even moving your lips. Alternatively, you may wish to listen to recorded music of this mantra.

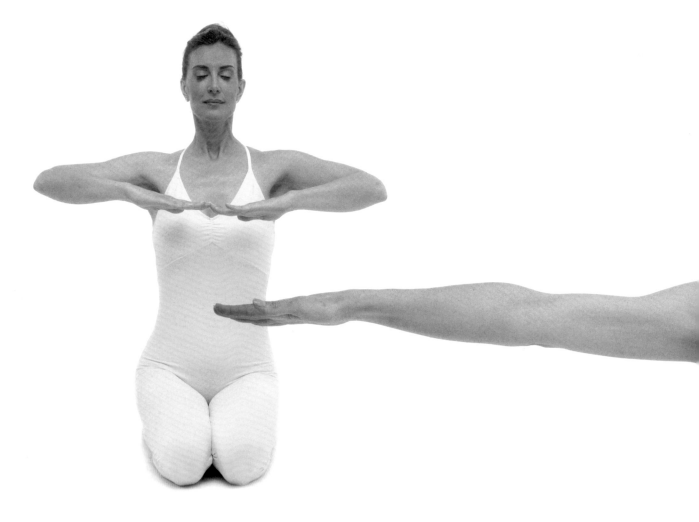

5 With each repetition of the mantra, slowly extend your hands out from your heart center straight to the sides, keeping your hands and forearms parallel to the ground and your palms facing down. As your hands move to the sides, powerfully pull in your abdomen at the navel, lifting the solar plexus and diaphragm slightly.

6 Move the hands and arms back into the original position with fingertips together in front of you, as described in step 2. Release and relax the navel as you bring the hands into center.

7 Repeat steps 5 and 6, continuing the arm movement while keeping your eyes focused at the tip of your nose and listening to the resonance of the mantra in your mind. Move the arms at a comfortable and consistent pace. Continue for three to eleven minutes.

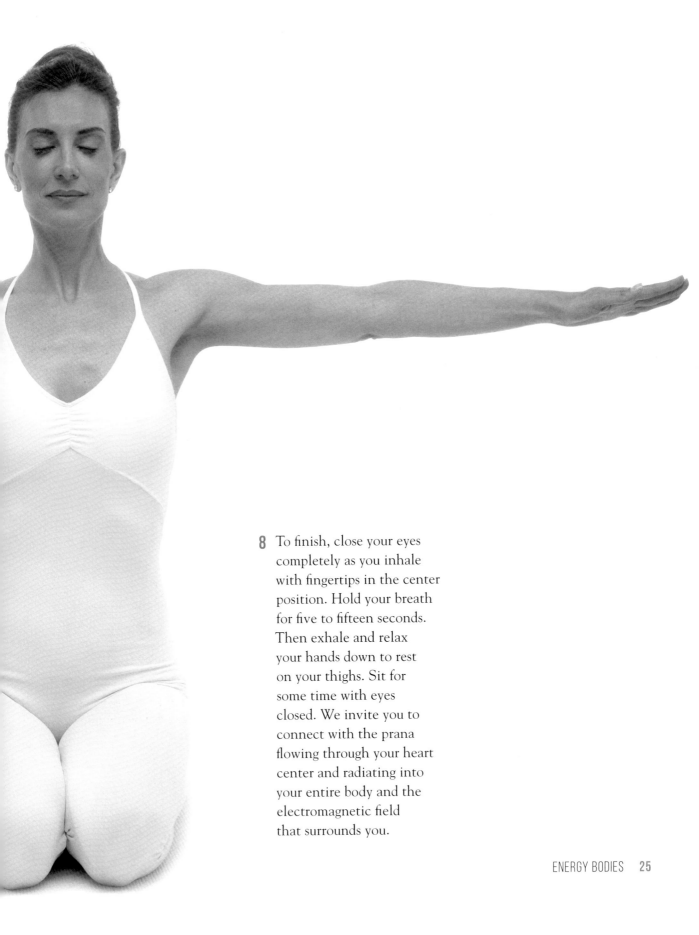

8   To finish, close your eyes completely as you inhale with fingertips in the center position. Hold your breath for five to fifteen seconds. Then exhale and relax your hands down to rest on your thighs. Sit for some time with eyes closed. We invite you to connect with the prana flowing through your heart center and radiating into your entire body and the electromagnetic field that surrounds you.

FIFTH CHAKRA: TRUTH

The fifth chakra corresponds to the throat, and holds the frequency from which we speak in our authentic voice. It is where impulse turns into choices and action in the world. In the physical body, this frequency is represented by the neck, the vocal chords, and the crossroads between the torso, head, and arms. The fifth chakra allows us to weigh our actions and make conscious choices about how we wish to communicate our authentic expressions that originate from our true self into the world. The color associated with this chakra is blue.

From the frequency of the fifth chakra, we verbalize, make sound, and do work with our hands and head. If this chakra is blocked, we may have difficulty expressing what is coming from our heart. When we put more effort into being polite to others than we put into being truthful to ourselves and the world, we create a very unbalanced fifth chakra. In essence, denying our truth will cause blockages in the fifth chakra.

○ YOGA FOR THE FIFTH CHAKRA CAMEL

Camel Pose balances the energy of the neck and throat and releases tightness there. This pose opens the entire throat and heart area, which enables us to love, give, and express without fear.

1 Kneel on the floor with your legs hip width apart and the thighs perpendicular to the floor. Relax your shins and the tops of your feet deeply into the floor. Place your palms on the back of your hips.

2 Inhale and lift your heart up while you allow your hips and thighs to press forward.

3 With your heart lifted, exhale and draw your shoulder blades toward each other to open the heart more.

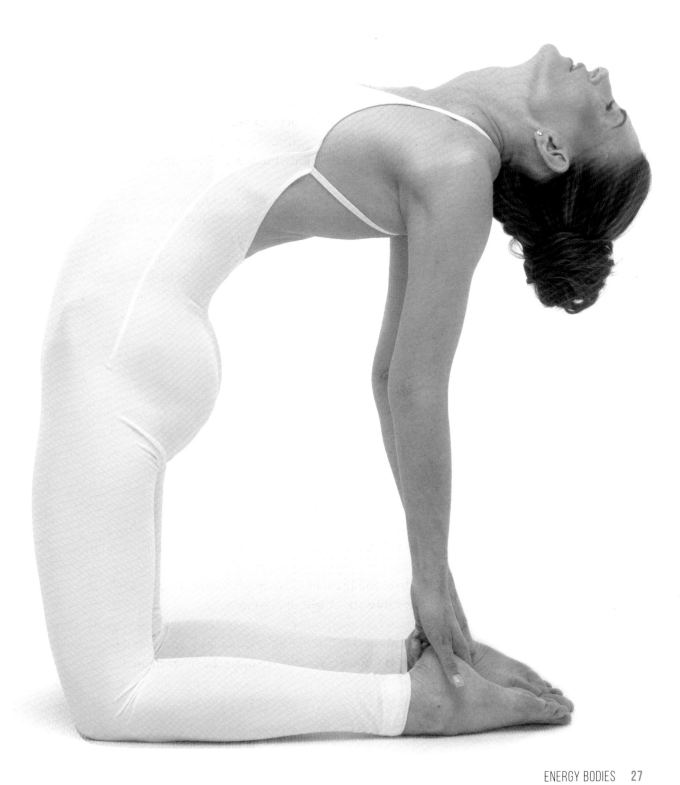

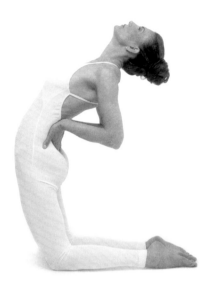

MODIFICATION If your hands do not touch your ankles, press your palms against the backs of your hips.

4 Breathing deeply in and out of your belly, continue moving your hips forward while gradually opening your sternum up toward the heavens. Pay close attention to the throat as you slowly lift your chin and tilt your head back.

5 Gently drop the head back as far as feels comfortable and lower your hands to your ankles. Continue breathing deeply.

6 Focus on relaxing your throat. Allow the healing energy in your throat to begin vibrating the sound "hummmmmmmmmm." on each exhalation. Release the sound out loud and continue for one to three minutes while holding Camel Pose.

7 To finish, inhale deeply, fully filling your lungs and gently holding your breath. As you exhale, slowly lift your head and gradually lower your hips back down until you are sitting on your heels. Give yourself the gift of time to sit, lie down, or come into baby pose, assimilating the effects of the posture and feeling the flow of breath.

SIXTH CHAKRA: INTUITION

The sixth chakra is a frequency of energy at the third eye, the seat of our intuition (or sixth sense). It physically corresponds to the point between the eyebrows, and its color is indigo. At its most basic level, the sixth chakra is sensitive to light and dark, day and night; from here the hormones for sleep and wakefulness are released. As we develop the sensitivity of the third eye, we become aware of very subtle shifts of prana, such as those caused by the feelings of others.

This sensitive awareness is our natural state of being. In the activated whole person, kundalini can flow freely to open or shut the third eye as needed in any given situation. When the third eye is balanced, we do not have to search outside ourselves for the answers. We simply know, intuitively, and we trust what we know as truth. We also realize that our wisdom is coming from our connection to the divine. When the fifth chakra is not balanced, however, we feel confused and have a difficult time making clear decisions.

○ YOGA FOR THE SIXTH CHAKRA GURU PRANAM

Guru Pranam is a powerful balancing exercise for our energy field. It is simple but incredibly transformative. The position is the body language of surrender, making the statement, both inwardly and outwardly, that "I bow and allow the flow of the divine." By holding the head below the heart, we create an energetic message saying that we are allowing the heart to lead the way. We sweep the pathway clear for divinity to enter and create an invitation within ourselves to receive. We remind the mind to release its grip and let the deeper, quieter wisdom of the heart to shine.

Placing your forehead upon the floor activates your intuition by bringing energy to your third eye point. The tipping of the head forward shifts cerebral blood flow, enhances the flow of cerebrospinal fluid, and activates the glow between the pituitary and pineal glands, releasing a nectar that helps prevent aging. When practicing the version described below, spread your knees and relax your shoulders so that your heart can melt downward.

1 Sit up on your heels in a kneeling position. Deepen your breathing and recognize the flow of your prana arriving with every inhale. Feel your spine elongate as you hold it up tall.

MODIFICATION If you have difficulty sitting on your heels, place folded blankets or firm pillows beneath your buttocks and straddle them with your legs.

MODIFICATION If your forehead will not go all the way to the ground, place folded blankets or firm pillows underneath your head as a support.

2 Spread your knees comfortably, hinge forward from your lower spine, and slowly move your navel toward the floor while extending your arms out toward the floor in front of you as well. Keep your spine elongated and move from the lower back until you can place your forehead on the ground in front of you.

3 Focus on releasing your lower spine toward the floor; then relax your entire back down toward the floor. Pay close attention to the vertebrae between your shoulder blades, melting that area so that your heart chakra can open.

4 Stretch your arms out on the floor in front of you and bring your palms together. Begin taking long, slow breaths, inhaling and exhaling fully while visualizing light all around you. Keep your palms together, pinkies lightly touching the floor, arms outstretched, and your whole body relaxed. Surrender to the pull of gravity. Settle into this position and continue to take long, deep breaths for three to eleven minutes.

5 We invite you to sweetly and gently press your forehead to the floor supporting you and toward the earth below you. This position activates meridian points that send messages to the pituitary gland, resulting in the release of hormones and neuropeptides that allow the mind to become peaceful and the intuition to speak.

6 To finish, place your palms on the floor to support your weight with your arms and then lift your torso, beginning with your lower spine. Slowly rise up, vertebra by vertebra, until your head comes up last. Take a moment before standing up or rest on your back for a few minutes before returning to your daily routine.

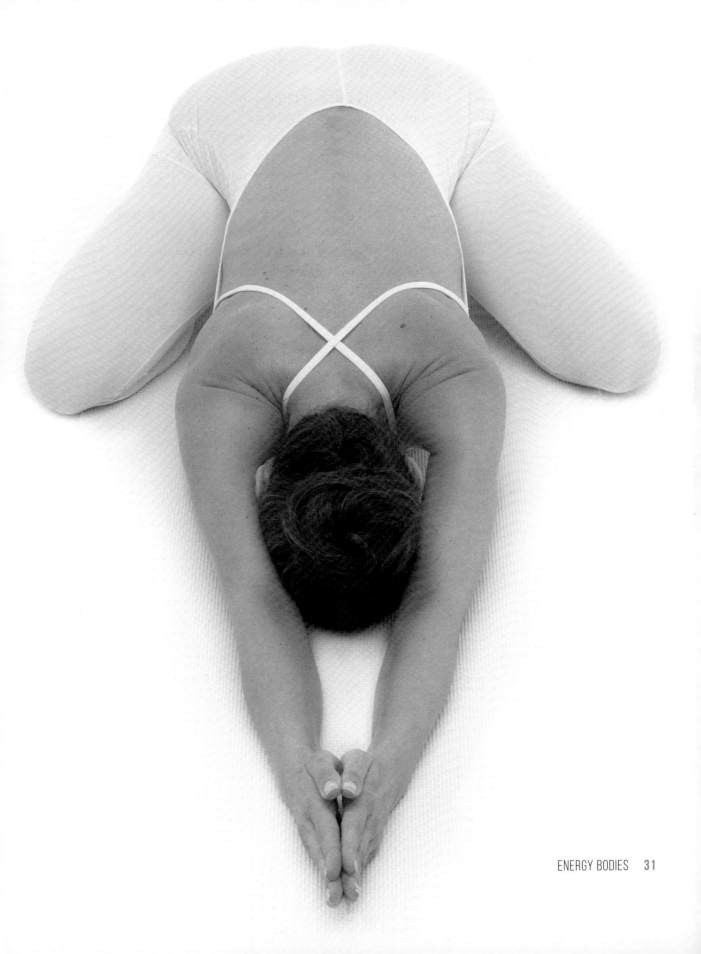

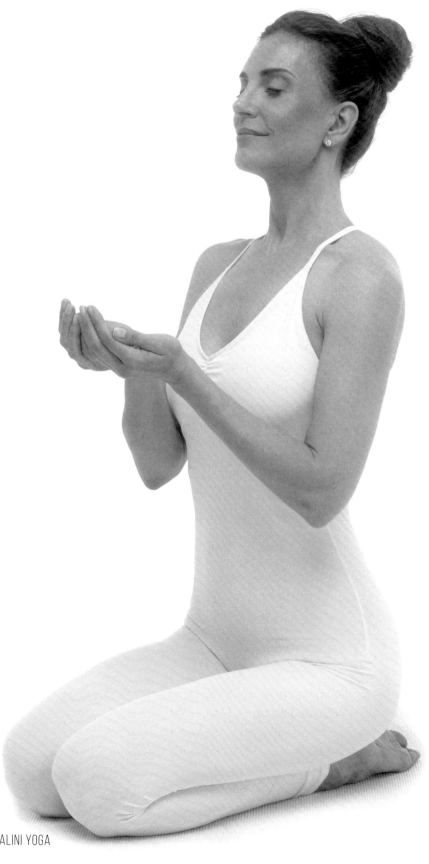

SEVENTH CHAKRA: GRACE

The seventh chakra is the energy pathway through which the pure prana of infinite wisdom merges with the individual nature of the soul. When we allow the flow of spirit to touch us at the seventh chakra, a new blossoming occurs in our consciousness. The seventh chakra, vibrating at the top of the head where the fontanel is, corresponds to the pineal gland. It is the gateway to angelic, love-infused prana. This is where we connect to spirit. Its color is violet.

Opening to the divine is a core part of the experience of being human. Everyone has this capability, but often, because of the way that religion has been misinterpreted, our experience of divinity comes weighed down with baggage, such as feelings of shame. Our innocent perception of God's ever-flowing presence becomes undermined by our thinking, rationalizing, and second-guessing. We start to feel small and separate, and we stop trusting our own experience. We forget that everything we encounter is part of a wondrous, loving consciousness that is coursing through us and breathing with us at this very moment.

Awareness that every sensation is a gift of the divine is called *Guru Prasad*. Guru Prasad is the reminder that we all are sparked by the same light and that we are part of the process of giving and receiving.

YOGA FOR THE SEVENTH CHAKRA
MEDITATION FOR GURU PRASAD

This fundamental and simple meditation opens us to the experience of our own connection with all there is. It bypasses all the trappings, the rules, and the limiting beliefs we might carry. All humans have the ability to simply experience their angelic nature, and Guru Prasad allows us to do that.

1 Sit on your heels in a kneeling position and feel your spinal column rising tall and filling up with the light of your soul. Give yourself time to breathe and to be present with the energy flowing through your breath.

2 Cup your hands together in a bowl shape, palms facing up toward the sky, in front of your heart. This creates a special kind of living bowl that receives light.

3 Relax your shoulders so your upper arms touch down snuggly but gently against the rib cage. Feel that you are in the presence of the divine and ready to receive a gift. Feel that the infinite universe is right with you, wanting to give gift after gift and blessing after blessing from its infinite abundance. Feel the universe pouring all these gifts into your hands for you to absorb into your being and into your life.

4 Lower your eyelids until your eyes are just barely open. Focus your vision on the tip of your nose. This focus opens the third eye and stimulates the optic nerve as it connects with the pineal gland. As this meditation progresses, however, feel free to close your eyes and focus internally on the third eye.

5 Begin long, deep breathing cycles, inhaling deeply through the nose and exhaling completely through the nose.

6 Open yourself to receive. Feel yourself being infused with the blessings of being part of a conscious, infinite universe. Allow the love of the universe to penetrate into your heart.

7 Continue for at least three minutes, but you are invited to keep going for as long as you like. So much joy and so much love are just waiting to enter you. Allow this vibration to resonate into every molecule of your body and into your aura. Open up, allow, and smile.

8 To finish the meditation, bring your arms down, place your hands in your lap, sit quietly, and resume normal breathing. Slowly open your eyes and see the world as a gift. As you rise and begin to move, feel yourself stepping into an energy field of delight, peace, and fulfillment.

EIGHTH CHAKRA: RADIANCE

Power is your presence.
YOGI BHAJAN

The electromagnetic field surrounding the physical body is our eighth chakra, which encompasses the totality of the resonance from all the other chakras. It is known as the *aura*. Just as white light combines all the colors of the rainbow into one, our eighth chakra combines all the frequencies of our being into one field. It extends as far as nine feet around our bodies and is extremely sensitive to the movement of energy, both from within us and from external sources. The color of this chakra is white.

We consider this the chakra of radiance because it radiates with a frequency that originates from the soul. Our inner glow becomes our outer glow by the projection of positive energy. When we say that someone has a healthy glow about them, we are intuitively referring to their radiance. Is our radiance a jumbled-up cacophony of disharmonious energy, or are we centered and clear? We can learn how to shift our radiance to one of health, vitality, and joy by aligning our vibration with the vibration of the infinite flowing through us. This is the key to manifesting a miraculous life.

When our radiance is aligned with our soul, our presence becomes our power. The love in our heart can ripple out through our body and flow into the world around us. We express confidence and attractive humility. We hold a magnetic grace around us. Our presence becomes our field of optimal possibilities, a magnet that draws bountiful, beautiful, and miraculous gifts. Our presence can even heal others.

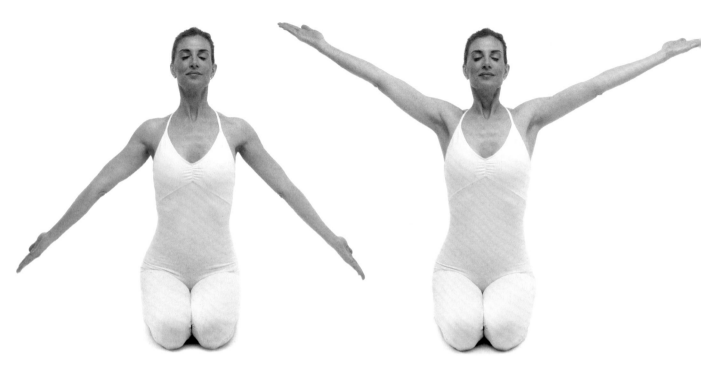

○ VISUALIZATION FOR THE EIGHTH CHAKRA
EXPAND YOUR ELECTROMAGNETIC FREQUENCY

Sat Nam

Everybody is a candle, but not everybody is lit. In this meditation you will be igniting the spark that the divine gave you. This meditation will give your skin a glow from the inside out. In this meditation we silently focus on the mantra "Sat Nam," imagining the sound rather than saying it out loud. (For more about this and other mantras, please see chapter 5.)

1 Sit with your spine straight, eyes closed, and hands resting in your lap. Gently roll your eyes upward and inward and focus your attention on the top of your head. Feel the flow of your breath.

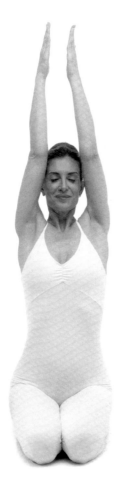
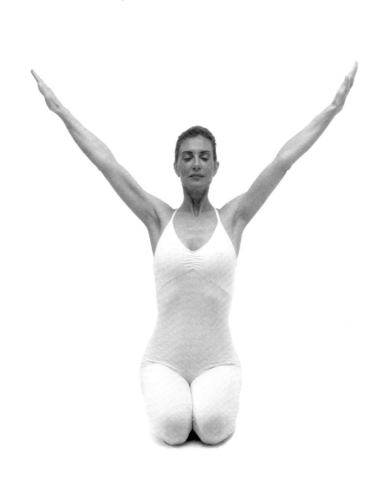

2 Imagine that you are a candle with a flame of light at the top of your head and a glow of white light that extends nine feet around you on all sides. Visualize it as a huge circle of illumination that radiates outward from your heart. Keep your eyes closed and looking upward upward and inward.

3 Inhale and slowly sweep your arms out and up, with your elbows straight, fingers extended, and your palms facing the sky. As you do, silently think of the mantra "Sat." In the long form, often used for meditation, the word *Sat* has a long, extended vowel sound that rhymes with the word *thought*.

Sat

4 At the end of the inhalation, keeping your elbows straight, touch your palms together overhead.

Nam

5 Once your palms touch above your head, turn the palms away from each other and slowly sweep the arms down as you fully exhale. Silently think of the mantra "Nam" as your arms sweep down. The word *Nam* is pronounced "naam" and rhymes with the word *calm*. Just think of that sound, without saying it.

6 As you sweep your arms down, visualize your hands clearing anything that is dense or heavy from your electromagnetic field. Think of light coming out from your fingertips as you sweep through this field.

7 Continue the arm movements and silently hearing the mantra for three to seven minutes. Feel that your inhale and exhale are leading the movement of the arms. You can choose any pace that feels comfortable.

8 To finish, inhale, lift the arms up, and hold the breath in. Exhale slowly, lower your arms one last time, and relax. Visualize the glowing energy of illumination within you and expanding into the space around you. Tune in to the extraordinary vibration that you have just created in your aura.

NADIS
YOUR ENERGY PATHWAYS

Prana flows through our body in a network of channels called *nadis* (pronounced "*nah*-dees"). The main channel of energy that flows from the base of our spine to the top of the head is called the *sushmana* (pronounced "*shoosh*-munn-ah"). In other yogic traditions it is also called the *shushmuna*. This pathway is revered as the conduit of our light and of kundalini.

Kundalini yoga works to keep this channel clear and vibrating with its core essence, love, so our energy can move freely, without blockages. As it does so we activate our higher potential as human beings. Although the sushmana follows the path of the spine, the nadis do not correspond directly to our physical anatomy. They are pure energy channels, sometimes described as threads of light.

Kundalini is concentrated energy, and as it rises through the shushmana, it activates each chakra and awakens our full potential. Kundalini yoga clears all the nadis and awakens our life-force so it can flow without restriction caused by our fears and insecurities. When awakened, kundalini flows through the central nadi, a new birth takes place, and love infuses its fragrance into our health, consciousness, and all of our life.

○ EXERCISE FOR CLEARING THE NADIS
ALTERNATE NOSTRIL BREATHING

This classic breathing exercise balances the flow of prana through the sushmana and the right and left hemispheres of the brain, clearing the pathway and creating a balanced integration of body, mind, emotions, and soul. Inhaling through the left nostril and exhaling through the right will assist you with anxiety, sadness, and anger. Inhaling through the right nostril and exhaling through the left will give you energy, clarity, focus, and stamina. By slowing the breath down and practicing alternately as described below, you will clear blockages in the nadis, develop intuition, and create a deep connection to the subtle energy flowing through all life.

While doing this breathing technique, slow your breath down as much as possible. Focusing on holding the breath in for as long as you can after the inhale and holding the breath out after the exhale. It is common to feel hot during this exercise as your vibratory frequency increases. It is also quite common to shake as your nadis release congested energy, especially if this practice is new to you. Those sensations will subside once your energy is flowing clearly. You are dissolving blocks and purifying toxins, and your body is adjusting.

1 Sit up tall and rest your left hand on your left knee, with the palm facing up.

2 Using your right hand, place your index and middle fingers on your forehead just above the ridge between your eyebrows. Close off your right nostril by pressing on the side of your nose with your right thumb.

3 Inhale as slowly and smoothly as possible through the left nostril.

4 Release the thumb and hold your breath for as long as you are able while imagining your prana circulating through your entire body.

5 Close your left nostril by pressing on the side of your nose with your ring finger. Gently exhale as slowly as possible through your right nostril.

6 Release the finger and hold your breath out for as long as you can.

7 Repeat the cycle for three to eleven minutes, alternating nostrils after each inhalation.

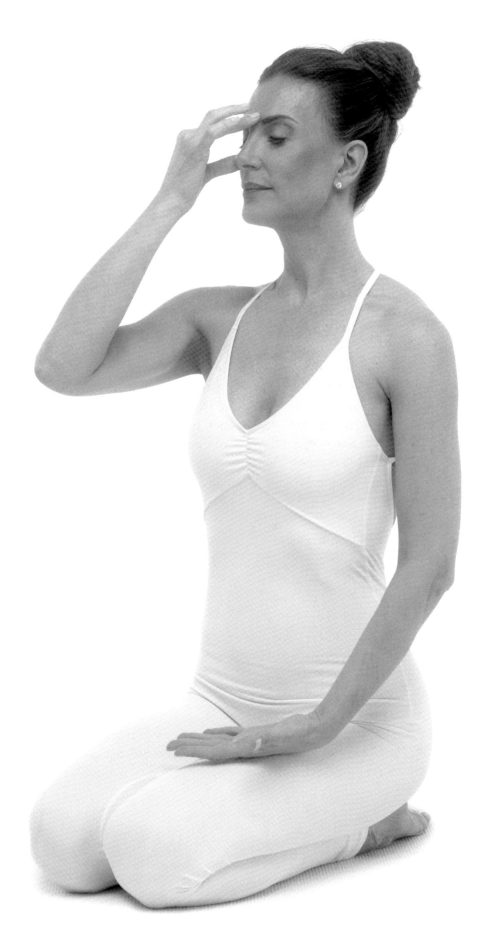

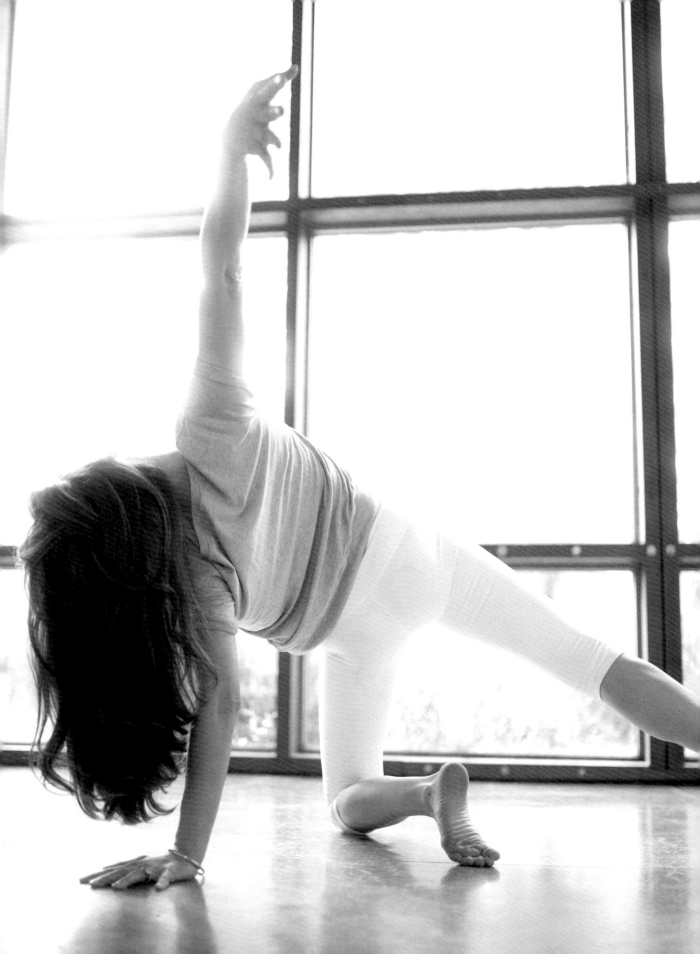

3 THE PHYSICAL BODY

Butterflies are not insects. They are self-propelled flowers.
ROBERT A. HEINLEIN

WHEN OUR PRANA MOVES FREELY through our physical body, we become alive with a compelling charm and a magnetism that attracts more positive energy. An exquisite series of physiological and emotional events takes place within our bodies, which we call the *health response*. Our bodies are electric, and just as electricity lines can have faulty circuits, our prana can lose its intensity. However, when the electricity of our physiology is flowing optimally, our prana radiates the most miraculous powers within our very own body. This is the purest form of vitality that is available to all.

It is our prana that enhances our physicality, making us healthy and radiant. Our thoughts, prayers, and attitude create an interaction of wave forms in our body that has a profound effect on us. Our well-being, our sense of happiness, our feelings of being loved, and our ability to give and receive love all depend on the activation of our prana. The most important attributes we have as human beings are actually the most subtle. It is our radiance, our flow, our grace, our intuition, our compassion, and our love that create the magnificence of who we are. The physical body is what we see; however, the attributes are what invigorate and heal the body from the inside out.

HORMONES AND THE HEALTH RESPONSE

Tiny shifts in our hormone levels can create massive changes in our personality. Most of us have experienced moments when our hormones are shouting and our soul is relegated to observing the reactions. Hormones can make us feel crazy at times, but they are also essential to awakening our brilliance. The ability to balance and enliven our endocrine system is a one of the fundamental breakthroughs of kundalini yoga. The breathing exercises, the pituitary gland yoga set in chapter 8, and many of the other exercises are like little miracles that move our hormones into a optimized state.

The pituitary gland is our master gland. It is the conductor of the orchestra in the symphony of our hormones. The pituitary delicately senses a myriad of functions, including input from the breath rate, hypothalamus, pineal gland, heartbeat, vibrational frequency, and our very own brain waves, especially our feelings of being loved. Conscious breathing, mantras, and thought patterns bring balance to our pituitary and entire endocrine system, in turn creating profound effects on our whole body, including our fertility, constitution, awareness, and energy levels.

Oxytocin is our love hormone. High levels correspond to feeling loved, trusting, and open to the deepest levels of intimate bonding, not only with others but also with the universe and with ourselves. Oxytocin soars during sex, cuddling, skin-to-skin contact, stimulation of the nipples, the sending and receiving of messages of love, and yoga practice. Under the influence of oxytocin, our breathing relaxes, our stress response subsides, inflammation lowers, and our genetic expression shifts. It is called the "love hormone," but could just as easily be called the "health hormone" because high levels of it are correlated with vitally healthy cellular response. The exercises we share throughout this book have helped bring many people back to a dynamic health response by activating their hormones and returning depleted oxytocin levels back to their natural state.

Hormones dictate our emotions, and our emotions can throw off our hormones. It is quite a vicious cycle, but kundalini yoga breathing techniques can interrupt the cycle and adjust our hormones back to a state of health. Fear makes us miserable. It pushes our hormones into an unbalanced state that was, in our cave person past, designed to enhance survival, but that unbalance wreaks havoc on our health, awareness, and ability to connect emotionally with others. When we are in fear, oxytocin plummets, adrenaline spikes, cortisol increases, and the signals from our pituitary gland generate a hormonal mix that activates the fight-or-flight response. We may notice that our breathing becomes rapid and shallow, our posture stiffens, and our voice wavers. Under feelings of panic our breath becomes impossible to control. In fact, the fear response also produces countless internal changes that go unseen, depleting our immunity, shortchanging our energy, scattering our focus, and reducing our life-span. The fear response is designed to save our life in short-term emergency situations; however, if it continues day after day, it will pave the way to dis-ease.

The magic of breath is that it reverses the effect. By controlling our breathing with techniques such as those described in this book, we dissolve the panic, actually shifting our hormones out of the fight-and-flight response and back into the health response.

The ancient practices of kundalini yoga revitalize our pituitary gland to orchestrate a positive health response. Our oxytocin levels increase, and we feel loving, whole, and connected again. When our hormones are balanced, the luminous flow of our prana unlocks, and we master the ability to transcend the mind.

THE PITUITARY AND PINEAL GLANDS

The pituitary gland is a small, pea-size organ located near the center of our brain, behind the bridge of the nose and above the back of the mouth. Medical scientists have discovered that it is in charge of the entire glandular system. The pituitary gland sends signals to the thyroid, adrenals, ovaries or testicles, heart, and lungs. It controls our entire metabolism, reproduction, blood pressure, endorphins, oxytocin, growth hormones, and many other hormones in the body. What the ancient yogis knew, however, is even more special: this little gland can be activated to create signals that open our consciousness to the awareness of our divine self.

The pineal gland secretes melatonin, helps us to relax, and opens our intuition. The space between the pituitary and the pineal gland corresponds to the third eye, which sees in a different way than our two physical eyes. The energetic line between the two glands—that radiance—was known to the ancient sages as the "golden cord." It is incredibly sensitive to changes in the magnetic field and especially to changes caused by other people's thoughts.

Slowing your breath down to less than one cycle per minute quickly activates the balance in the pituitary and pineal glands. By practicing the breathing technique below, you can generate clear intuition while creating an optimal balance in your hormonal system.

Square Breath is our favorite breathing exercise. Many doctors and psychologists teach this breathing technique to clients because it is easy for everyone to learn and practice. It is called Square Breath because it has four equal parts.

○ SQUARE BREATH

1 Sit up in a cross-legged position with your spine straight. Rest your palms comfortably on your knees, facing upward. Close your eyes and focus your attention on the third eye point.

2 Tune in to the flow of breath entering your nostrils and filling your lungs. Feel the breath as a light that is alive and is loving you.

3 Inhale as slowly as possible to a count of eight, feeling the energy of your breath. Take the breath in deeply, allowing your diaphragm to descend into your abdomen and completely filling every portion of your lungs.

4 Hold your breath for a count of eight.

5 Exhale as slowly as possible to a count of eight.

6 Hold your breath out for a count of eight.

7 Repeat the breathing pattern, making the count slower and slower with each round. You can adjust the pace of the count to work with your lung capacity. To slow down the breath, simply count to eight more slowly. Another variation is to count along with your heartbeat.

THE NERVOUS SYSTEM

The sensory system that will develop automatically out of us will be our archangel protecting us and glorifying us.
YOGI BHAJAN

The parasympathetic and sympathetic nervous systems—also known as the PNS and SNS—are the two systems that hold our entire sensory system in balance. The SNS awakens, and the PNS soothes. One is like a roller coaster; the other is like a chaise lounge. Humans have a profound ability to use opposites, but this ability works only when our nervous system is regulated and balanced. Ever notice that if you push too hard, things do not work out? Or if you offer no resistance when you know it needs to be applied, you are not able get beyond a block? Physiologically these experiences are determined by the balance between the two nervous systems.

The SNS energizes our survival response. Whether triggered by an approaching tiger in our cave person evolutionary past or by an angry boss stalking down the hall today, the effect of the fight-or-flight reaction on our body is the same: ligaments tighten, adrenaline flows into the bloodstream, the organs become restricted, breath rate increases, digestion is inhibited, and the ability to fall asleep is often disturbed.

The PNS acts like a breath of fresh air. Its signals tell our body to relax, loosen up, enjoy the moment, sprawl out, get comfortable, smell the roses, and breathe deeply. Our heart rate slows down, blood pressure lowers, our skin glows, we lose weight, our digestion

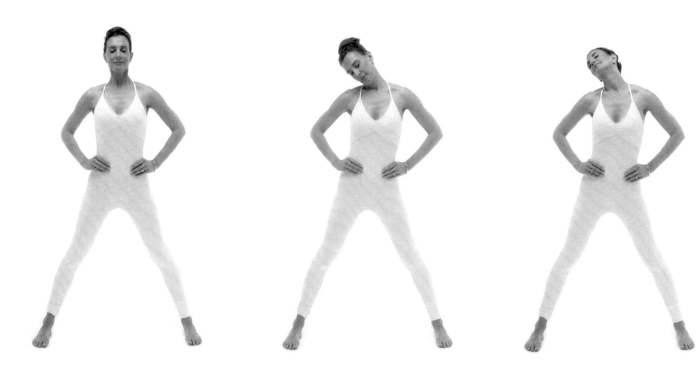

improves, our cells begin to repair themselves, and our mood is happy. We can enjoy the people and things around us.

Yoga and meditation are some of the very best ways to stimulate the PNS so that it balances the SNA; these techniques can help us use the two opposing systems to hold our consciousness in harmony. Thank God for these practices in the high-stress world in which we live.

○ YOGA FOR BALANCING THE NERVOUS SYSTEMS

Neural pathways at the base of the spine and the neck regulate the PNS. By relaxing our neck and jaw while bringing energy into the lowest part of our spine, we can activate the remarkable power of the PNS, bringing a state of calm and feelings of love back into our life. A basic tool to remember is this: when you feel stress in your body, do an exercise to relax your neck and lower back and activate your PNS. Simple neck rolls at your desk or hip rolls can act like magic. You can use these two simple movements anytime and anywhere to turn down your stress response and return to the peaceful, functioning, creative sense of self that is at your core.

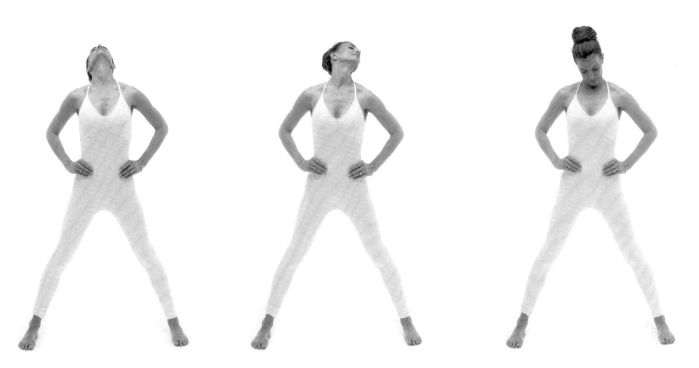

THORACIC NERVE STIMULATION

1 Stand up tall with a straight spine, shoulders relaxed, feet in a wide stance about three feet apart, and hands on your hips. Feel a line of energy connecting your navel to mother earth below you. Your feet are rooted firmly into the floor. Allow your jaw to relax and drop slightly open, feeling the pull of gravity.

2 Begin to take long, slow breaths, drawing the breath so deeply into your body that you feel it pressing into your sex organs.

3 Drop your chin down toward your chest. Begin gently rotating your head and neck, making wide, unhurried circles. As you inhale, slowly rotate your head out over your left shoulder. Keep rotating your chin up toward the sky and tilting your head all the way back as you finish your inhalation. As you exhale, continue rotating your chin down toward your right shoulder and, finally, back toward the center of your chest as you complete your exhalation.

4 Repeat the movements and breathing pattern, going very slowly and allowing yourself to really feel the stretch in the many muscles that run through your neck. Continue for three to twenty-six rotations in the same direction.

5 Reverse directions and repeat the same number of times as in step 3. This will balance the left and right hemispheres of the brain.

6 To finish, hold your neck up straight, inhale, hold your breath in, and then exhale and relax.

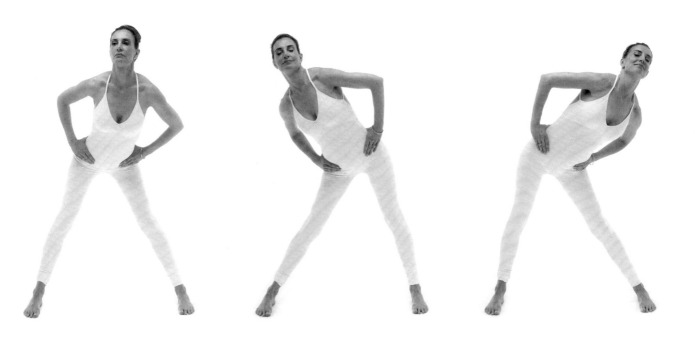

○ SACRAL NERVE ACTIVATION

1 Keeping your stance wide and your hands on your hips, as in the previous exercise, begin rotating your pelvis in wide horizontal circles. Inhale as you circle forward and exhale as you circle back. Pay attention to flexing your lower spine. Continue for one to three minutes.

2 To finish, inhale, bring your pelvis to center, stand tall, hold your breath in, and hold this posture for a moment. Then relax and feel great. Tune in to the sense of calm and safety that activating the parasympathetic nervous system gives you.

The vagus nerve is a pathway of nerves carrying messages back and forth between brain and body that affect our heart rate, breathing, voice, digestion, sexuality, and many other functions. New science is showing that the vagus nerve is also the main conduit for the messages of love. The body tells the brain to release oxytocin by sending signals through the vagus nerve. When the right signal flows through the vagus nerve, our pituitary releases more oxytocin, and voilà: love, love, love.

Vagus nerve stimulation boosts neurotransmitters that help us to feel calm, confident, and secure. Using a treatment approved by the FDA in 2005, doctors have been treating depression, seizures, and eating disorders with electrical stimulation of the vagus nerve. In kundalini yoga, rather than electrodes, we use ancient, time-tested exercises to optimize the flow of prana through the vagus nerve. We don't have to depend on the ebb and flow of external conditions in order to be in love. We can experience the love vibrating within our own being. It is there all the time.

○ WHISTLING BREATH FOR THE VAGUS NERVE

Whistling Breath increases vitality, clarity, relaxation, and our sense of comfort and well-being. It acts on the vagus nerve by stimulating the biofeedback loop from the diaphragm to the midbrain. This breath can bring the physiological system into a beautiful state of calmness. It can actually lower cortisol levels, which aids in weight loss. Did you know that you can lose weight by utilizing effective deep breathing techniques? Well, you can.

This is also a great exercise to do when you have a craving to consume something unhealthy. If you find comfort in food when you feel depressed or anxious, practice this exercise and see if you feel a decrease in cravings.

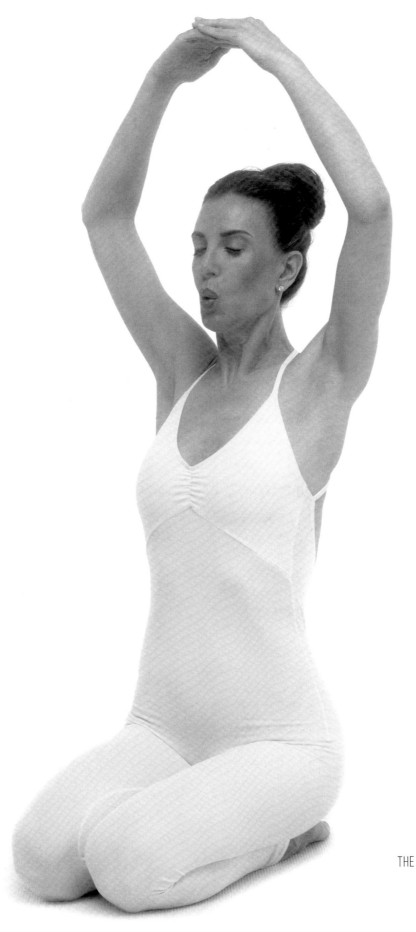

1 Sit with your arms lifted into a circle, both hands about six inches over your head, with your palms facing down and your left hand over the right.

2 Put your lips together and whistle as you both inhale and exhale, fully filling and emptying your lungs. Make your whistle as long and steady as possible, feeling your consciousness merging into the sound. Continue for three to eleven minutes. If you can't make an actual whistling sound, the technique is equally effective if you pucker your lips and breathe through them as though you're whistling. The action of the lips in a whistling position is directly correlated to vagus nerve stimulation.

3 To finish, inhale deeply and hold your breath. Exhale, bring your arms down, and sit with the shift in your consciousness.

CEREBROSPINAL FLUID

Cerebrospinal fluid (CSF) is like a constantly circulating river that completely bathes our brain and spinal column. When it is fresh, it is a delightful source of life, but when polluted, it toxifies all that it touches. If it is not circulating well, our mind becomes foggy and our body sluggish.

We are continually creating and exchanging our CSF at an incredible rate—up to five pints per day. There is recent evidence that the incomplete clearing of metabolic wastes, such as beta-amyloids, generates early biomarkers of Alzheimer's disease as well as other diseases. The incomplete circulation of CSF may bring on many aspects of aging itself.

In addition to washing away wastes, CSF delivers essential vitamins, hormones, and nutrients to the brain. It carries the love hormones, oxytocin and vasopressin, to their receptors. This delivery system boosts our ability to fall in love and to feel loved in natural ways. Yogis have known for thousands of years that this clear, almost luminous liquid is the stuff of life.

The key to keeping CSF fresh and alive is movement. We do not circulate CSF efficiently without movement. When we are sedentary for long periods of time, our body can start to develop stagnant areas that reabsorb old toxins. Kundalini yoga deeply and profoundly renews the CSF around our spinal column and brain, keeping us bright and alert, like a mountain river. The yoga practices will clear the waters of your body and bring sparkle and purity back into you.

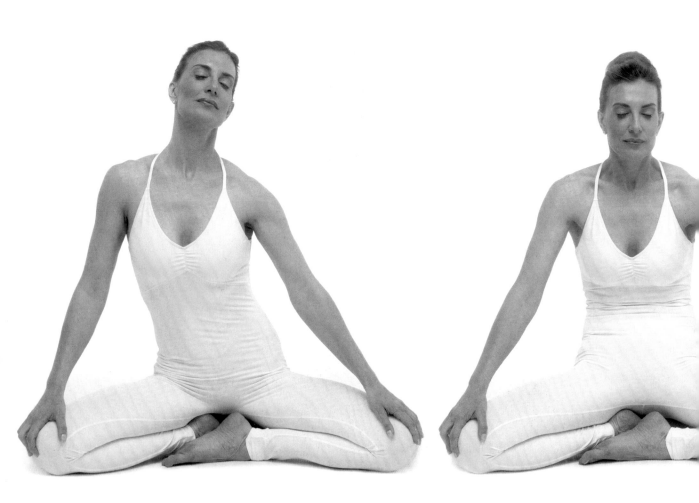

○ THE DIVINE GRIND

It is quite amazing how easily a simple kundalini yoga exercise can keep our cerebrospinal fluid healthy and alive. This is an exercise that many can perform. It is a great practice to do before and after long car or airplane rides. It is also very beneficial if you have been in bed for a long time.

1 Sitting in a crossed-legged position, breathe deeply and connect with the source of all life flowing through you. Close your eyes and go deeply within. Visualize the flow of energy through the central channel of your spine.

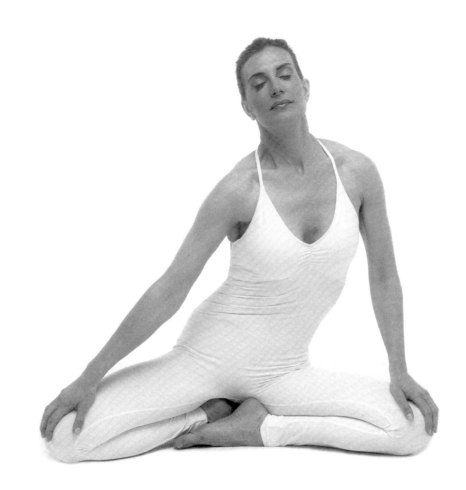

2 Place your palms face down on your knees. From the base of the spine, begin rotating your lower spine in circles, keeping the shoulders straight but relaxed. Inhale as your spine flexes forward and to the side, and exhale as you arch back and around to the other side. Your rib cage and abdomen will be expanding with the inhalation and compressing during the exhalation. Continue in one direction for twenty-six or more circles and then reverse the direction and repeat for the same amount of time.

3 To finish, inhale deeply as you bring your body to the center, with your spine rising tall between your pelvis and top of your head. Stop the movement and hold your breath. Exhale and relax your entire body. Finally, resume normal breathing.

RADIANT HEALTH
ENERGY AND OUR GENETIC POTENTIAL

The purified, integrated mind, so perfected in its own
understanding, lives in close communion with the soul radiance
so that light becomes the constant companion of the mind.
SIVAYA SUBRAMUNIYASWAMI

By uplifting our vibrational frequency and activating the flow of kundalini energy, we create frequencies in our electromagnetic field that awaken new possibilities for genetic expression. An amazing vastness of genetic potential is coded into our DNA, but it is often not accessed because we have not yet created the bioelectric environment required for its expression. The vibrational environment that a cell divides within is shifted by our thought patterns. Until our magnetic field reaches the vibrational frequency required for a given gene to express its potential will remain unexpressed. The essential frequency that unlocks our genetic potential for resounding health and clarity of consciousness is the frequency we call "love."

The *placebo effect* has shown scientists for decades that thoughts and emotions have the power to change the way our cells express their genetic potential. The placebo is a little sugar pill used in experiments that contains "nothing" medicinal, but because our mind thinks it is "something," our cells actually divide differently. In other words, because of what we think, wounds seal together, broken bones fuse, and organs reactivate, all because of shifts in activity at the genetic level. Our genetic expression depends on our thinking because our thinking changes the vibration of our energy field.

There is so much more coded into DNA than has been expressed so far in our human evolutionary development. Each cell is highly sensitized to a vibrational picture being created by the entirety of our being. In other words, genetic expression—our health and our happiness—depends on what we think and what we do. A 2015 study found that 90 percent of disease is caused by environmental and energetic factors. Only 10 percent of disease is genetically rooted.

Fulfilling our genetic potential is a natural drive, like the drives for food, warmth, and companionship. In this era, many of us are feeling called to surpass our limitations—the limitations of our family's concepts, the limitations of our self-concepts. If you are reading this book, most likely you have felt this calling. Often we have no models in the modern world for what we know in our hearts to be the potential that we can achieve. We are the explorers of our inner world. Unfortunately, while toxicity and diseases are prevalent everywhere, so many of the health imbalances today are caused by repressing the soul's yearning. However, we blame the imbalances on illnesses that we have caught or toxins in our foods. Have you ever felt out of alignment, upset, or completely exhausted after spending time doing something that you did not agree with? Have you ever caught an awful cold after spending a weekend with someone who drained all your energy? If you are saying yes to this, we encourage you to listen to the voice in your heart so you can get better and better every single day.

○ YOGA FOR HEALTH VITALITY STRETCH

The ancient yogis taught that the flexibility and flow of energy through what they called the *life nerve* determined our health and life-span. The life nerve is actually a long bundle of nerve cells extending from the lower spine through the buttocks, down the back of the legs, calves, and heels, and out to the toes; its pathway corresponds to that of the sciatic nerve and major energetic pathways. We know today that the individual nerve cells can be several feet in length and the bundle as thick as a garden hose. The condition of these giant nerve cells powerfully affects our entire constitution. When the energy flowing through our life nerve is blocked, the fibers themselves can become inflamed, and our entire constitution feels constricted. The following exercise is excellent for opening up the flow of energy through the life nerve, boosting the immune system, and healing the body from a basic cold, bug, or flu. It is highly beneficial for everyone to practice daily.

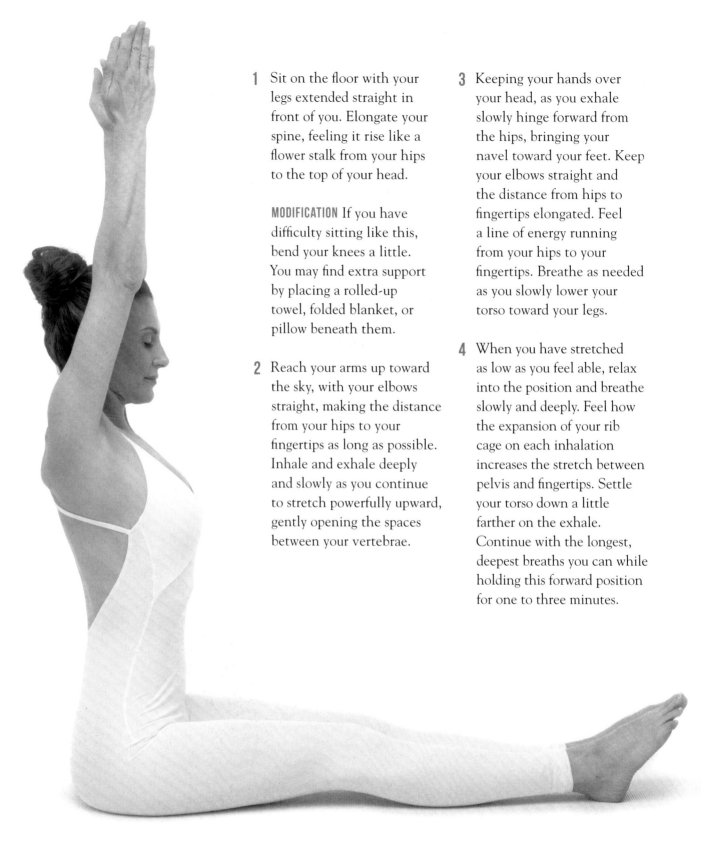

1 Sit on the floor with your legs extended straight in front of you. Elongate your spine, feeling it rise like a flower stalk from your hips to the top of your head.

MODIFICATION If you have difficulty sitting like this, bend your knees a little. You may find extra support by placing a rolled-up towel, folded blanket, or pillow beneath them.

2 Reach your arms up toward the sky, with your elbows straight, making the distance from your hips to your fingertips as long as possible. Inhale and exhale deeply and slowly as you continue to stretch powerfully upward, gently opening the spaces between your vertebrae.

3 Keeping your hands over your head, as you exhale slowly hinge forward from the hips, bringing your navel toward your feet. Keep your elbows straight and the distance from hips to fingertips elongated. Feel a line of energy running from your hips to your fingertips. Breathe as needed as you slowly lower your torso toward your legs.

4 When you have stretched as low as you feel able, relax into the position and breathe slowly and deeply. Feel how the expansion of your rib cage on each inhalation increases the stretch between pelvis and fingertips. Settle your torso down a little farther on the exhale. Continue with the longest, deepest breaths you can while holding this forward position for one to three minutes.

5 Inhale and lift your torso back upright, with arms still raised, to the position in step 2. Exhale and hinge down forward again. Stay focused and present with the action; do not go fast.

6 Leading with your breath, keep the up-and-down movement going with a steady rhythm, inhaling as you come up and exhaling as you fold your navel toward your thighs. Each time you extend upward, inhale and imagine filling yourself with positive energy. As you fold over the legs, exhale and imagine letting go of any negative energy. Continue for up to twenty-six repetitions.

7 To finish, inhale, come up, and hold your breath. Exhale as you hinge fully forward, then hold your breath out. Repeat two more times, ending in the upright position.

8 Resume your normal breathing and sit with the energy you have created, sensing the flow of prana in and around you.

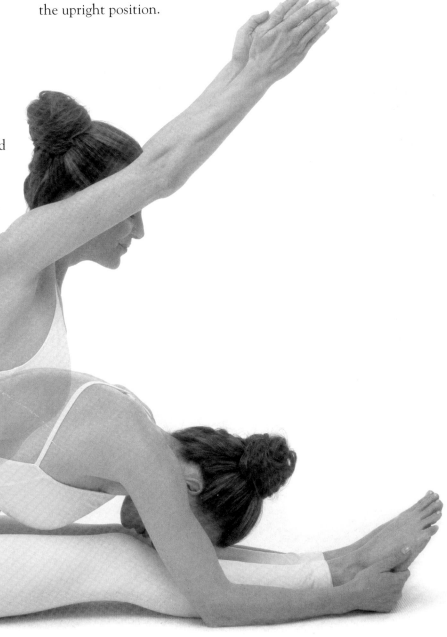

UNLOCKING OUR GENETIC POTENTIAL

Everything we think and feel resonates in and around us in our electromagnetic field. DNA is acutely sensitive to the frequency of its electromagnetic environment. When DNA operates within an electromagnetic environment of the highest frequency, which is love, it can express in miraculous ways that the courser frequencies of fear, anger, and competition simply do not allow. If you see DNA when its strands are extracted from a cell nucleus, it appears to collect light, glistening like an optic fiber. Kundalini yoga tunes our electromagnetic field to reach the frequencies required for our full genetic expression.

The quest of our life is to let that true brilliance of our being shine. When we release the inner blockages, the energy of our soul can penetrate into the physical environment of our body and surroundings. The more we give up our own restrictions, the closer we become to the pure energy, the pure love, that beams out from our source. It is time to step out from the cave that hides our light. It shifts our very genetic nature when we do so.

There is an energetic field around our physical body that literally emits light. While this field is generally not visible to the physical eyes, it is so powerful that when it is balanced and healed, it can rebuild the physical body. This is also the field that makes a person attractive to another person. We do not need to dress in fine clothes or wear mascara to activate the electromagnetic field. Simply sitting and vibrating in the frequency of all-encompassing love is more than enough—and it is free. The magnetic field is the field that draws all successful endeavors to us, and it actually controls our personal strength, clarity, and vitality.

MAGNETIZING YOUR ELECTROMAGNETIC FIELD

The electromagnetic field, also called the aura and the eighth chakra, is the field of possibilities that surrounds the physical body. When we are clear of blocks in our electromagnetic field, our radiance vibrates outward into the atomic structure all around us like rays of sunshine. Yogis have used the principle of sympathetic resonance for thousands of years to create what some consider to be miracles. The vibration that we create in our own electromagnetic field will resonate into the world around us. The vibration in this field becomes a magnet for similar vibrations in the world. This is why we say, "Be grateful, and you will receive more of what you are grateful for."

When our radiance from the field around us is activated, unbelievable opportunities arrive without the physical body having to work in the usual sense. We can sit and vibrate and let the blessings come, thanks to the clarity of our electromagnetic field.

When we plug into the divine, focus on gratitude, give to others what we desire, live for the highest good of all, allow our heart to lead us, meditate to quiet the chatter of the mind, and release the limiting belief systems from our childhood and ancestral lineage, our aura expands and attracts naturally. The shift begins in our electromagnetic energy field. There is much fascinating beauty in this field, and every single person who walks this earth has the potential to activate it. What a miracle this is.

A ripe manifesting potential arrives when we activate our electromagnetic energy field by surrendering to the grace of the infinite. We can do this with our personal practice of elevating our energy frequency. The energy that surrounds our body holds a force that we often just do not tap into. Once you realize the magnitude of this field, your life can change in magnificent ways. It is so important at this time that we recognize the sensitivity of the magnetic field. There are environmental disturbances in this field that we cannot always control, for example, from cell phones and Wi-Fi. We urge you to put your cell phone on airplane mode and turn your Wi-Fi off at night when you are sleeping. Also, surround yourself with plants as much as possible to purify the negative charge from the electromagnetic field.

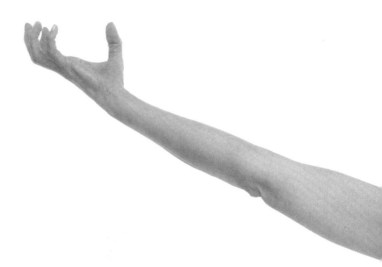

○ THE LION CLAW EXERCISE
TO RESET YOUR ELECTROMAGNETIC ENERGY FIELD

This powerful exercise clears the electromagnetic field around our physical body. Think of Lion Claw as a way to clear toxins from the energy egg that is around you while also working the physical body.

The arm movement energizes the nervous and lymphatic systems and awakens the pineal gland, so your radiance can project more powerfully from your electromagnetic field. This is one of our favorite exercises for clearing our energy field and allowing our potential to shine brightly.

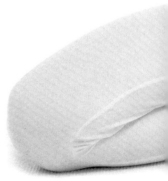

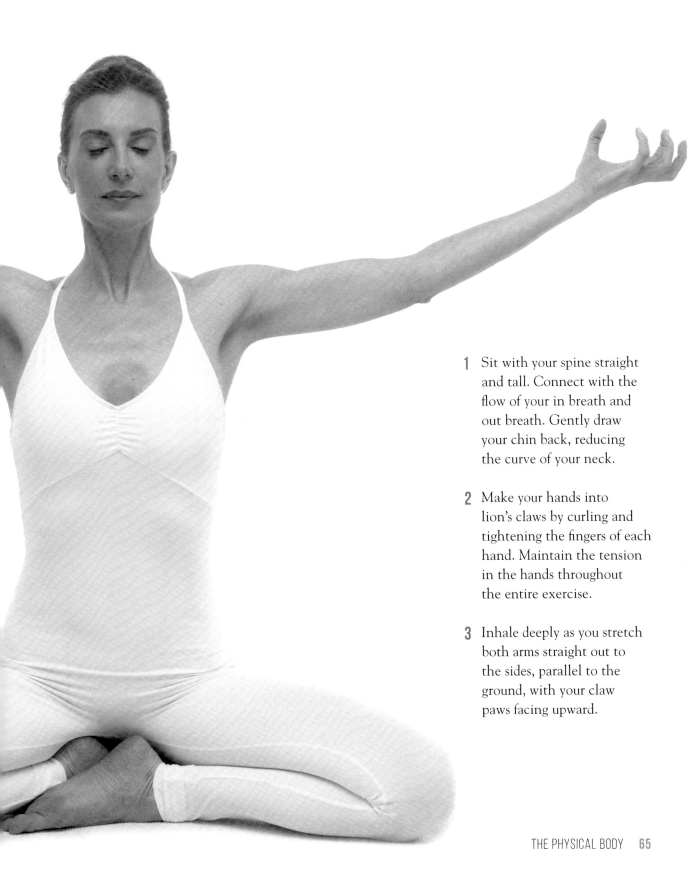

1 Sit with your spine straight and tall. Connect with the flow of your in breath and out breath. Gently draw your chin back, reducing the curve of your neck.

2 Make your hands into lion's claws by curling and tightening the fingers of each hand. Maintain the tension in the hands throughout the entire exercise.

3 Inhale deeply as you stretch both arms straight out to the sides, parallel to the ground, with your claw paws facing upward.

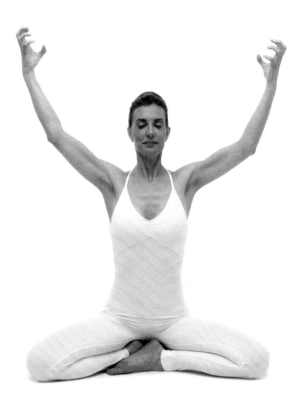 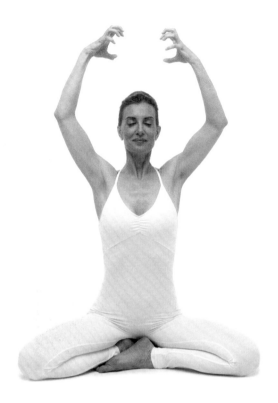

4 Exhale and swing your arms up overhead and slightly forward so that your hands crisscross each other above your forehead and the palms end up curving down toward your head.

5 Inhale and bring your hands back to the starting position in step 3, with arms out to the sides.

6 Repeat the movement, allowing your breath to direct the motion. Alternate one wrist crossing in front, then the other. Continue with a rapid motion for one to nine minutes.

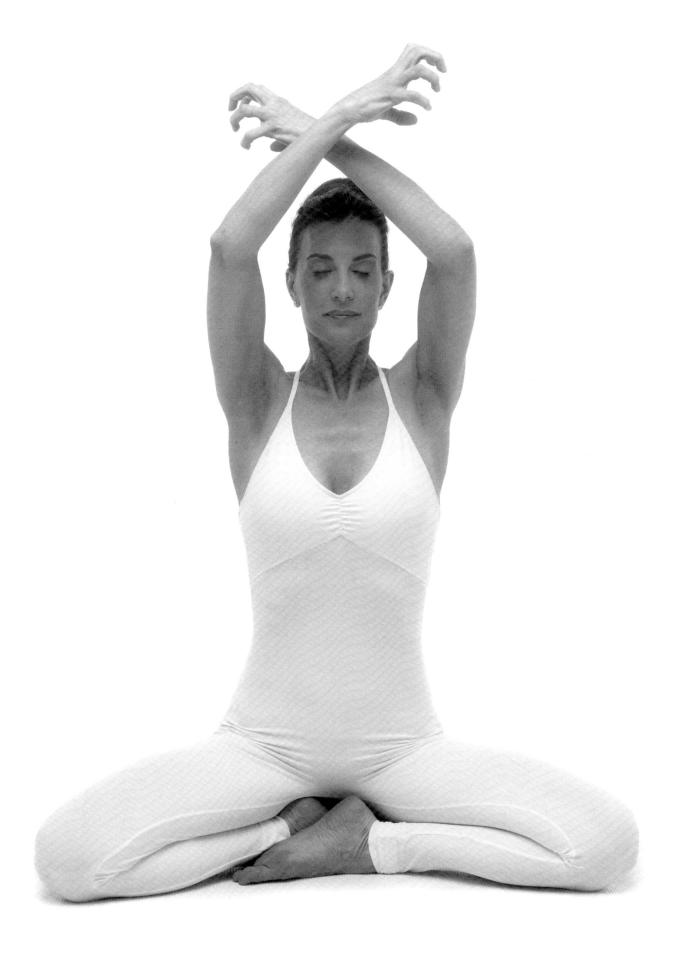

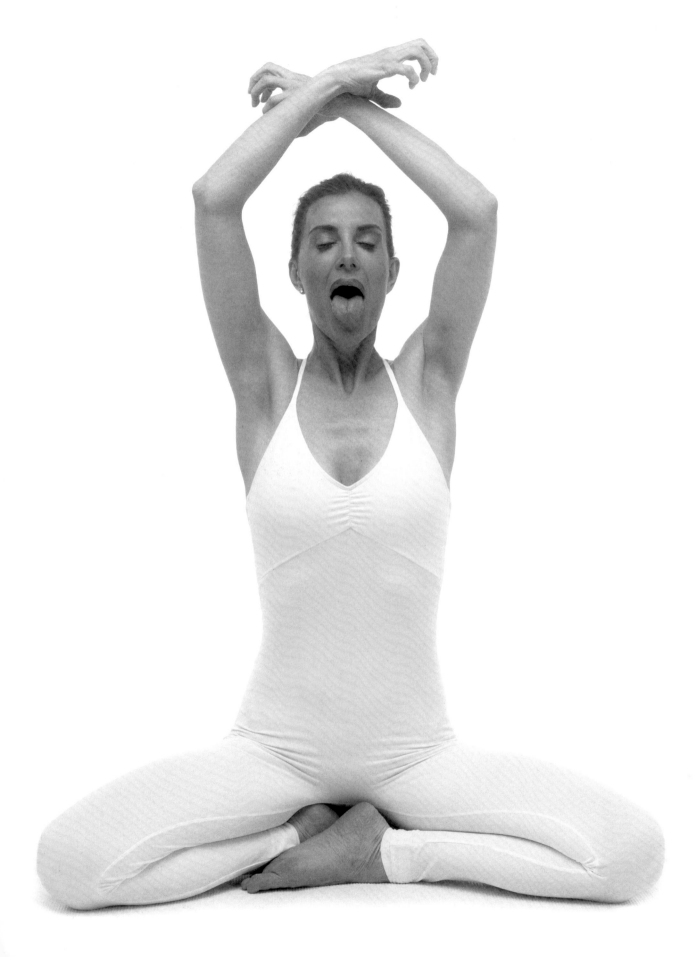

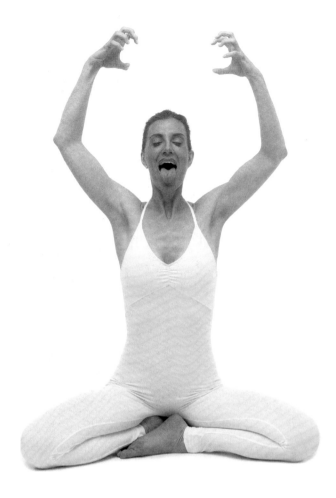

7 Now open your mouth, stretch your tongue out and down, and continue the motion while breathing through the mouth for fifteen more seconds.

8 Keep your mouth open and tongue stretched out and down. Maintain the claw grip, but now stretch your arms overhead and outward at a sixty-degree angle as you exhale your breath completely and forcefully from your lungs. Hold your breath out as long as you can, for up to fifteen seconds.

9 With the arms and tongue in the same position, inhale deeply and hold the breath in for thirty seconds.

10 Exhale slowly and consciously through your nose as you relax your arms down, allowing your breath to come back to normal. Breathe freely and feel the flow of energy through your magnetic field within and around you.

11 Continue to breathe as slowly and deeply as possible. We invite you to feel grateful for this opportunity to clear your electromagnetic energy field of anything toxic, uplift your frequency, and attract to you the beautiful blessings that arrive when we are in alignment with spirit. You have just created a potent field that can manifest the infinite possibilities available. Enjoy it. Sit with your eyes closed and whisper, "Thank you."

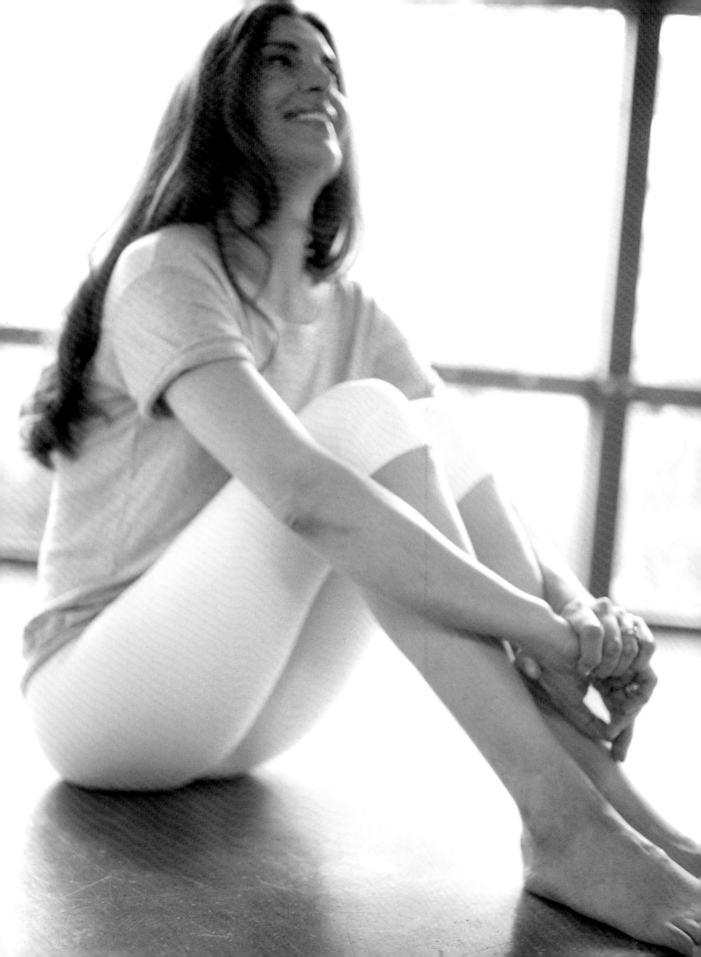

4 BREATHING FOR TRANSFORMATION

When the pranic bodies are augmented, all bodies are
perfectly in order. Because between you and God
there is only one link and that is the breath.
YOGI BHAJAN

WE WOULD LIKE YOU TO release the concept that you are breathing air and embrace the concept that you are breathing light. Envision light pouring through the spaces between the atoms of your body. Search for where that light is not penetrating in your body and in your life. Absorb the light, via the breath, and direct it with your mind to wherever you feel it is needed. What you bring attention to becomes energized. If there is one thing you take away from this book, may it be the importance of using the breath to bring balance to your mind, your body, and your life. As we affect the breathing, we affect our ability to absorb the energy of love.

Deep and expansive breathing makes us calm and generates physiological health benefits, such as reduced blood pressure, increased focus, and weight loss. It can be practiced anywhere—while you are eating consciously, waiting in line, flying or riding for long periods of time, finding patience in a chaotic situation, or performing any form of exercise. We encourage you to return to your breathing whenever you remember to throughout your day, not just in a yoga session. Stay connected to the subtle yet most divine gift of breath.

YOUR DIAPHRAGM

The diaphragm is like an inverted, flexible bowl that extends across the inside of your torso at the level of your bottom ribs. We like to think of it as being a trampoline. It can be pulled down into the abdomen, drawing air into the lungs. It can be pushed up toward the ribs, expelling the air from the lungs. Because of the resilience of the tendons that it is constructed of, it has a natural resting point that it returns to. Tune in to your diaphragm and see if you can discover its neutral resting point when it is being neither pushed nor pulled.

KUNDALINI BREATHING TECHNIQUES

In yoga, the breath has four parts to be aware of: the inhale; the moment we can hold our breath in after the inhale; the exhale; and the moment we can hold our breath out after the exhale. The holding is called *suspending the breath*. All four parts of the breath are important, but we tend to overlook the magical moments of suspension. In kundalini yoga we pay special attention to the times you hold your breath in and hold it out. This is when energy circulates, our resistances dissolve, new pathways emerge, and miracles happen.

At the very end of a kundalini exercise there is a beautiful opportunity to inhale, suspend the breath, and connect with the oneness of the universe. All the work we have done during an exercise leads up to this crystallizing moment. Often we suspend the breath several times, holding on the inhale as well as on the exhale. Give yourself time and allow this sacred moment to penetrate to your depths.

We are passionate about the breathing exercises in kundalini yoga, and we urge you to practice one or all of the techniques we share below. Deep breathing is one of those powerful secrets that our world does not discuss much. If everyone understood the potency of these breathing exercises, our world would change for the better in profound and beautiful ways.

○ BREATH OF FIRE

Breath of Fire is the signature breathing technique of kundalini yoga. It charges the cells, vacuums impurities out the energy pathways through the body, stimulates molecular exchange through the lungs, strengthens the nervous system, purifies the blood, energizes and brightens the aura, balances the hormones, speeds up the metabolism, and aids in the release of toxins. Via the vagus nerve, Breath of Fire also creates a biofeedback loop that generates deep inner stillness and the ability to focus. It creates a sacred and magical heat that can burn away stubborn wounds. It is the magic breath.

In our experience, the easiest way to learn Breath of Fire is by starting with an open mouth, but once you get the hang of it, do it with the mouth closed.

1 Begin by lying comfortably on your back with your legs extended. Allow your diaphragm to relax completely and come to its neutral resting point.

2 Open your mouth and began panting like a puppy on a hot day. Breathe out in short, forceful exhalations at a speed of two to three breaths per second, allowing your lungs to take in air in between. With each exhalation, pull the navel back sharply and push the diaphragm up toward the ribs to expel the breath.

MODIFICATION. You may bend your knees or place a rolled-up towel, folded blanket, or cushion behind your knees to be more comfortable and to reduce strain.

The inhalation is created by relaxing and letting your diaphragm do the work. If you focus on making a steady, rhythmic series of exhales while pushing the diaphragm upward, the inhales will automatically happen during the moments in between, and they will balance the volume and rhythm of the exhalations.

3 Once you have the rhythm, close your mouth while you keep the breath moving steadily. Continue breathing through your nose at the same speed as you were panting before. You may continue for as long as you like.

4 To finish, inhale deeply, hold your breath in, then gently release it and breathe normally. Feel the shift in your energy level.

At first it may feel as though your whole body is struggling to figure out Breath of Fire. See if you can relax and allow the breath to move. If you watch experienced practitioners, their spine stays almost completely still, and only the abdominal muscles move with the signature rapid pumping. With just a bit of ongoing practice, it becomes easier and easier to isolate the core muscles of the abdomen. Breath of Fire will become your friend, energizing and purifying your nervous system.

Typically Breath of Fire is practiced for several minutes, although sometimes longer. It is often done while one is holding various yoga positions and occasionally in conjunction with movement. It can be practiced as a seated meditation for up to half an hour. Once you have the muscles working properly, it is soothing, centering, calming, and invigorating all at the same time. It speeds up the metabolism and gives a beautiful glow to the skin. This is one of the best-kept beauty secrets of kundalini yoga. You can observe this for yourself. Look in the mirror and then close your eyes and practice Breath of Fire for three minutes. Open your eyes and look at yourself in the mirror again. You will appear refreshed, and your skin and eyes will have a new sparkle.

○ SEGMENTED BREATH

Segmented Breath opens our intuition and sensitivity. Breaking the breath up into a series of sniffs, rather than taking one long, deep inhalation, stimulates and balances the endocrine system. For thousands of years yogis have used this practice to create hormonal balance, clear the mind, and bring vitality to the nervous system. The segmented inhalation is a reset button for the pituitary gland, optimizing its impact on all the other glands in the body, and the action of each sniff also has an enlivening effect on the radiance of the pineal gland.

The following is an eight-part Segmented Breath. You can do this while seated, but it is also a wonderful technique to practice while walking outside.

1 Sit up straight and tall, with your hands resting on your knees. Tune in to the sensation of breathing through your nose and the expansion and contraction of your rib cage. Feel the motion of your diaphragm as you draw air deeply into your lungs.

2 When you are still and ready, divide your inhale into eight equal sniffs. It may take several repetitions to get the length of the sniffs right so that the lungs are just as full after eight sniffs as they are after one long inhalation. Once your lungs are full, hold your breath in and let the prana circulate.

3 When you are ready, consciously, slowly, smoothly, and beautifully release the breath through the nose in one long inhalation. Holding your lungs empty for a moment, feel the energy circulating within you. Consciously register your posture, the emptiness of your lungs, and the pure prana as it moves through your body.

4 Repeat the inhalation, holding, exhalation, and holding cycle for three to eleven minutes.

5   To finish, inhale deeply, hold your breath as long as you like, and then release it slowly. Tune in to the shift in your energy as you resume normal breathing. You may wish to sit for some time.

○ BREATH FOR INTUITION

This breathing technique combines Segmented Breath, which activates the golden cord of radiance between the pituitary and pineal glands, with O-shaped lips, which stimulate the vagus nerve. This breath awakens the radiance of the pituitary and pineal glands, sensitizing our response to subtle shifts in the magnetic field in and around us.

1   Sit up straight, breathe, and feel your presence on the earth.

2   Bring your palms together in front of your chin and interlace your fingers, with the index fingers extending straight up and the thumbs crossed.

3   Gently lower your eyelids until they are almost closed and focus your gaze at the tips of your fingers through your almost-closed eyes.

4   Make your lips into an O shape.

5   Inhale powerfully through your mouth in four equal segments, each about a second long, so that by the end of the final segment your lungs are completely filled. With the lungs full, hold the breath suspended and feel the energy of that breath circulating through your being.

6   With all the awareness you can bring, close your mouth and exhale slowly through your nose in one long exhalation. Hold your breath out until you are ready to inhale.

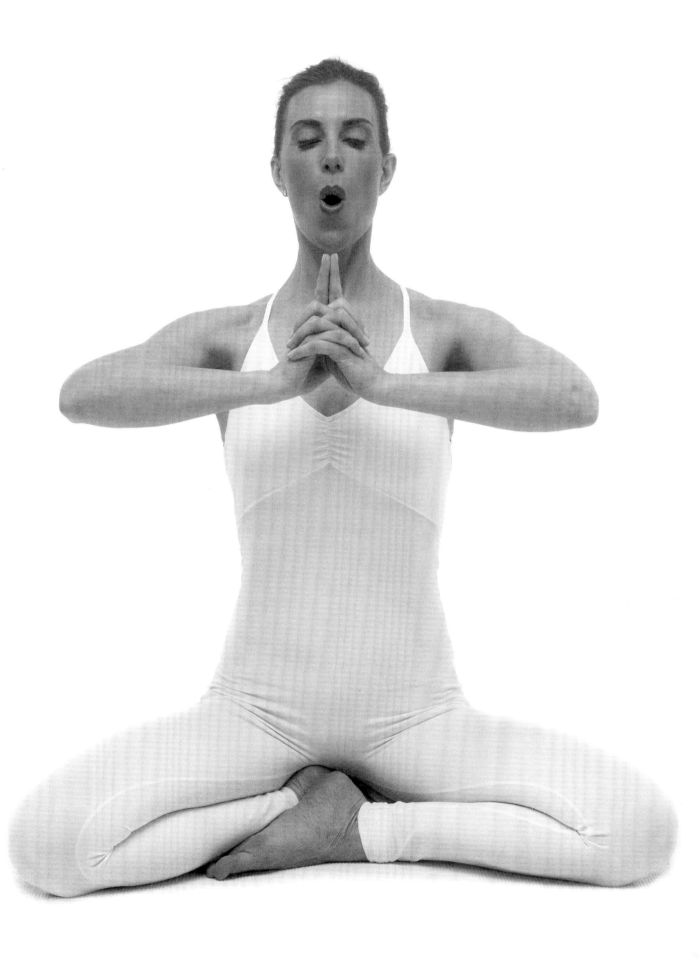

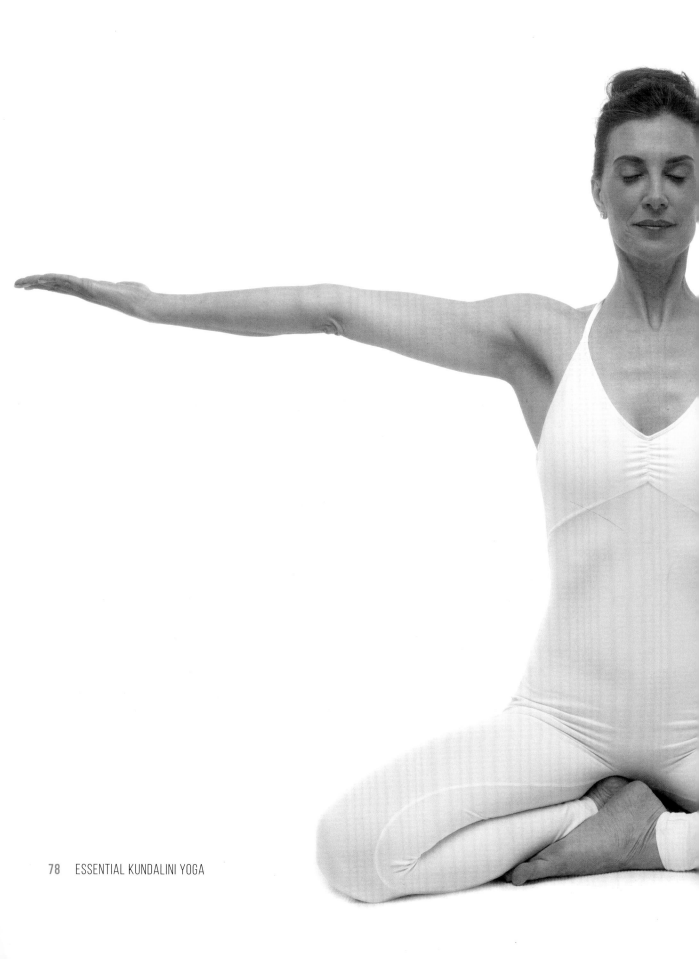

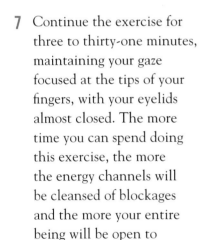

7 Continue the exercise for three to thirty-one minutes, maintaining your gaze focused at the tips of your fingers, with your eyelids almost closed. The more time you can spend doing this exercise, the more the energy channels will be cleansed of blockages and the more your entire being will be open to the flow of fresh prana.

8 To finish, with your spine straight and tall, straighten your elbows and stretch your arms out to either side, parallel to the ground, with the palms facing up. Pushing your fingertips outward, stiffen your fingers and feel the energy flowing from one palm through your heart to the other palm. Make your fingers as stiff and strong as possible.

9 Maintaining the position, inhale deeply through your nose and hold your breath in for up to twenty seconds. Exhale. Repeat the cycle, focusing all your concentration on your third eye point.

10 To close the practice, close your eyes completely, relax your arms down, breathe softly and normally, and continue to sit in silence to sense the effects. When you feel you are ready to do so, open your eyes.

○ MIRACLE BREATH

Miracle Breath is our all-time favorite breathing exercise. This breath uses the lips and tongue to create a powerful effect on the brain stem that helps you be in control of your own prana. It activates the pituitary gland, which allows us to directly experience our vastness and our ability to cocreate with the infinite on earth. It is based on an ancient technique from the oldest historic writings of yoga. We hear from people who say that this breath changed their lives in astounding ways.

Underneath the joy and the inspirations, the hurt and the disappointments, the strivings and the reactions, there is a river of love, constant, flowing like luminescent liquid light, alive and aware of you and me. We can cocreate with that river, respond to its call to participate in creating love. When we consciously choose to agree with our worth as a person, with love and trust and without ego, the dam floodgates open, the waters flow freely, and the self rises up and starts flourishing with magnificent beauty.

1 Sit in a cross-legged position with your eyes closed. Place your palms face up on your knees. Begin breathing deeply and slowly, allowing your inhalation to touch the base of your spine and the exhalation to reach to the top of your head.

2 Pucker your lips, making the center of your mouth as small as a pinhole and positioning the tip of your tongue right behind the pinhole. As you draw in your breath through your puckered lips, direct a cold stream of air to hit the very tip of your tongue. Consciously pull the diaphragm down into the abdomen as you inhale.

The key to Miracle Breath is to pucker so much that you create a resistance to the airflow while expanding the diaphragm. This greatly strengthens the diaphragm and lungs. Breathe steadily and calmly but powerfully at the same time, feeling the cool stream of air hit the tip of your tongue.

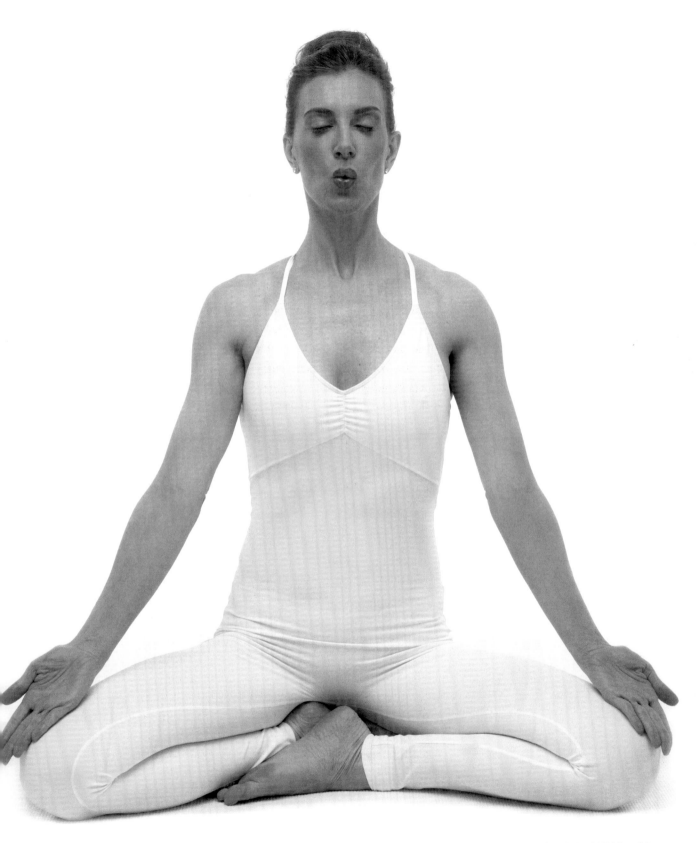

3   Once you have inhaled completely, close your lips, hold your breath, and move the tip of your tongue so that it touches the highest point of the upper palate. Press your tongue gently yet firmly against the roof of your mouth as you calmly hold the breath in for as long as you feel able.

4   When you are ready to exhale, let the breath escape as slowly as you possibly can through the nose. Take your time so the breath emerges in a steady, slow stream.

5   Once the breath is fully out, again calmly suspend the breath for as long as you are comfortably able. As you get more used to the practice, your pituitary will start to secrete in an enhanced state and you will find you can extend the time that you hold the breath out.

6   Repeat steps 2 through 5 for one to five minutes.

7   Follow with Breath of Fire for sixty seconds.

8   Continue alternating Miracle Breath and Breath of Fire for one to five more cycles.

9   To finish, complete your last round of Miracle Breath. Then inhale deeply, place the tongue against the roof of your mouth, and hold your breath in. Exhale slowly through the nose and hold the breath out. Then slowly inhale and breathe normally.

10 Sit quietly for as long as you can to allow the practice to assimilate into your being.

5 THE MIRACLE OF SOUND AND MANTRA

I do not just believe in miracles, I rely on them.
YOGI BHAJAN

WHAT IF YOU HAD A way to instantly counteract the negativity that crosses into your life? What if you had a way to bring joy and centeredness into your mind as simply as throwing a switch? What if you had a way to release your mind from the spiraling whirlpool of thoughts and instead could really feel the clear, open goodness of God flowing through your entire being?

Sound can permeate our beings, our physical bodies, our emotions, and our spirit. Sound penetrates through walls, through air, through our brains, and through our consciousness. When the sounds we create are heard in the next room, we are manifesting ourselves in that space. Loud sounds can create tension, and soft singing can create peace. Our inner being is carried a great distance with the use of sound.

The power of sound can shatter the restrictions that we may have built around our true self. The term *glass ceiling* implies a limit that is unseen but prevents advancement. We create a personal glass ceiling in our consciousness when we do not trust that the divine is working with us. But think of the stories of opera singers breaking glass with the vibratory power of their high notes. Doctors use sound waves to shatter kidney stones in a procedure called *extracorporeal shock wave lithotripsy.*

In a similar way, sound can break you free of the inner mental structures that limit you from raising your vibration into your fullest expression. Sound shatters the opacities that prevent your inner diamond from shining. Conscious use of sound is perhaps the most powerful way to access the river of love that flows through our being at all times.

The simplest, quickest, and most powerful way to create this inner shift is with the chanting of mantra, which transforms the sacred wisdom of sound into healing. Mantra creates a frequency that reminds us to flow with the river of love and surrender into peace. Mantra enables us to stop pushing and swimming upstream. Mantra allows possibilities to emerge without strain. We become a magnet, attracting the same vibration that we harmonize with through sympathetic resonance.

Think of long nails scraping slowly across a blackboard and hear that strange, screechy sound in your mind. Chances are you will have goose bumps, perhaps even right now just from reading this. This demonstrates how a simple thought or even a memory can create a powerful physiological effect. Sound always carries a mood, and that mood also changes our physiology. The vibrations of a sad song flowing through our nerves make us stop, breathe deeply, and think of a lost love. Similarly, when we create sacred sound, we infuse our vibration with the beauty of the divine. This process opens blocks and delivers us into the grace of our own consciousness.

While screeching sounds are usually short-lived, the sound of our own words can create powerful effects that comfort or hurt, and the imprint can last for many years. The words we choose can uplift, or they can cut like a knife, making scars that never heal. What we say and how we say it become our destiny fulfilled. We imprint the world around us, and we imprint our own beings. We have been gifted with the beautiful power and awesome responsibility of consciously choosing the sounds we deliver into the world. Speaking words and tones of love will attract the same sound vibrations of love. This is the law of the spoken word.

PRONOUNCING SACRED SOUNDS

In this book, we want to get you started with the power of chanting so you can begin to experience the beneficial effects of these ancient mantras right away. The mantras in the kundalini tradition are intended to be universal and support anyone's faith or belief, no matter what it is.

You do not need to consider yourself a singer to chant mantras. Simply allow your voice to express outward into the light body that surrounds you. It has nothing to do with "sounding good." The mantras can be expressed in a monotone or set to melodies. The sounds are simply a tool to vibrate into your body and electromagnetic field, and they will do the work. Opening your mouth and allowing sacred sounds to vibrate from you is chanting. Chanting is more about intention, expression, and devotion than it is about staying on key.

We have endeavored to make the pronunciations as simple as possible with English phonetic equivalents. Two simple nuances are important to be aware of as you read the pronunciation of the mantras. The first is that the R in kundalini yoga mantras is always pronounced like a soft D. The R is rolled once, so the tip of your tongue touches lightly on your upper palate. That delicate touch of the tongue to the upper palate is essential because it stimulates the pituitary gland, which is situated above the roof of the mouth. The second is that when you see a double "aa" in this book, it means the sound "ah."

MANTRAS

Mantras are sounds with a coded vibration of positive energy that connect our mind with the universal grace of our soul. When we express a mantra with love, the sound current carries that love into our own being and out to the world around us, vibrating the molecules of the physical environment that surrounds us. It can purify our consciousness, uplift our spirit, and heal our body. Our thoughts are energy patterns, and the energy pattern generated by a mantra enhances our thoughts naturally.

Mantras create an energy pattern inside our body that unlocks the expression of unique, life-giving neuropeptides and neurotransmitters. As the tongue taps the roof of the mouth, we stimulate the hypothalamus and pituitary gland, which has the power to balance our entire glandular and energetic systems. The rear lobe of the pituitary gland begins its development from the upper palate, and touching the tongue there opens an almost direct gateway to the pituitary. When the awakened physiological effect is combined with the emotion of divine grace, it unlocks the doorways to genetic expression and clarity of mind that allow our soul's light to shine brightly into our lives. This is what makes the kundalini mantras so life changing.

An easy way to think of mantra in our modern world is to compare it to a cell phone. We dial specific numbers on our phones to reach a certain person. The numbers create a sequence that extends out into energy waves, and the one specific phone on the other side of the waves is reached. The sounds of a mantra are like the numbers on the phone. They are chanted in a specific sequence to reach a certain outcome. It may seem to be a miracle that the sounds of "Ra Ma Da Sa" have healed people all over the world. However, years ago, if someone had said a little piece of metal would have numbers that could be pressed to reach another piece of metal across the world, or that two little devices would be able to exchange vibration, sounds, frequency, words, and even love from one soul to another, we might not have believed it. One day we may see that mantra is scientifically explicable as well as miraculous.

○ MEDITATION ON THE PRIMAL SOUND "MA"

One of the most ancient syllables for meditation is "Ma." In many cultures "Ma" means "mother." We start by vibrating our closed lips on "mmm" and open the resonance in our midbrain on the "aaa." The sound "maaa" resonates into the body with great power and calms the nerves while connecting us with the living wisdom of sound itself.

Ma

The mantra "Ma" is very healing. When chanting this mantra, you can feel as though you are calling out to your mother to help you. The mother energy is also the energy of the earth and the love you long for. Allow your expression to be free with this mantra. Allow your feelings to release. Dig deep inside and liberate yourself from pain and yearning.

1 Lie comfortably on your back with your hands on your belly. Breathe deeply and completely, feeling your abdomen rise and fall with each breath.

2 Begin humming on the exhale, making an "mmmm" sound, penetrating all your awareness into the sound. Sensitize yourself to the vibration, feeling everything about it—in your lips, tongue, teeth, roof of the mouth, and skull, but also in your spine, ribs, shoulders, hips, legs, and abdomen. Feel your vocal chords vibrating and breath emerging through your nose.

3 Notice, now, that you can direct the vibration of the humming internally to whatever area within your body, thoughts, or energy field needs healing. Continue chanting while using your sensitivity to feel the sound and direct it where needed. Change the pitch as you like to be most effective.

4 Now add the sound "aa," creating the full sound of "Ma." Think of an intention you would like the sound to carry with it, such as healing, gratitude, compassion, or love.

5 Feel the vibration flowing not only within your body but into your external environment as well. It touches the air around you, changing the air. Then the air penetrates the walls and furniture, trees and sky. Notice how the vibration can be directed in the external world with your attention. Now you have combined raw sound, attention, and intention to make an exceptionally potent force.

6 Feel the vibration shift from your lips to your midbrain. Continue the steps as before, making the sound into a healing medicine for you, for your environment. Feel that you can direct the healing to anyone you think of with the power of your attention. Observe the feelings and sensations that come through your awareness and your body. Continue chanting in this way for three to eleven minutes.

7 When you are finished, allow the energy of silence to bathe you like a soft mist. Sometimes the mantra "Ma" brings tears because it reminds us of being children and feeling the nurturing energy of the mother.

THE SEED MANTRA, "SAT NAM"

Sat Nam   The most fundamental mantra in kundalini yoga is called the Seed Mantra: "Sat Nam." If you learn only one mantra, "Sat Nam" (pronounced "*sutt* naam") is the one to learn. A vibration more than actual words, "Sat Nam" penetrates deep inside our soul to nurture the seed of our intentions. This is how the latent possibilities of consciousness sprout and grow. Just as a seed contains the blueprint of a giant oak tree, this mantra contains the blueprint of timeless awareness. Just as a seed will grow from darkness toward light, this mantra will activate a beauty from deep inside that grows into the form of your fullest divine potential, your true self. *Sat Nam* means "the name of truth." *Sat* means the timeless, all-encompassing truth, and *Nam* means "name" or "identity." We are all manifestations of truth in the depth of our soul. From the affirmation "Sat Nam" our awakened consciousness can flourish, and we can live our lives with harmony.

You may vibrate "Sat Nam" silently or chant it out loud. When we repeat a mantra silently, the mantra lights up the same pathways of the brain that chanting aloud does. In kundalini yoga, we often vibrate the mantra during an exercise that coordinates with our deep breathing. On the inhale, imagine the word "Sat" becoming a silent sound that vibrates up the spine to the ethers. On the exhale, imagine the word "Nam" becoming a silent sound that brings the spiritual manifestation of light into the earth realm. The Seed Mantra is one of the most powerful meditations we know.

○ LONG "SAT NAM"

For this variation of "Sat Nam," extend the length of the first syllable to become a very long "Saaaaaat," using almost all your exhalation. Chant a short "Nam" at the end, as follows.

1   Sit up straight, feeling the flow of prana through your body. Place your hands together in Prayer Pose at the sternum.

2   Inhale deeply. As you chant "Sat," exhale and feel the vibration rising up through the central column of the spine, starting from the very base of your spine and ascending to the very top of your skull. The wisdom of sound is ascending through your spine and clearing the path.

3   Almost at the end of your exhale, when you come to the delicate, sharp *t* made by an exquisite touch of the tongue against the upper palate, feel the vibration of that *t* unlocking the gateway to the universe at the very top of your skull.

4   With the final portion of the same breath, allow the word "Nam" to resonate through your vocal chords and radiate into your electromagnetic field. Imagine the sound expanding into your environment as a manifestation of light.

5   Take another long, slow, conscious inhalation deeply into your belly. Chant the mantra again as in steps 2 to 4. Continue chanting for three to thirty-one minutes. As you do so, observe the sacred sound of truth vibrating inside and filling your spine with light. Set an intention and spend this time knowing that the seed you are planting with your intention is sprouting.

6   When you are finished, allow the "mmm" sound at the end of the "Nam" to penetrate into your heart. This "mmm" sound will nourish the seed of your intention. Relax and experience your connection to the wonder of the miraculous.

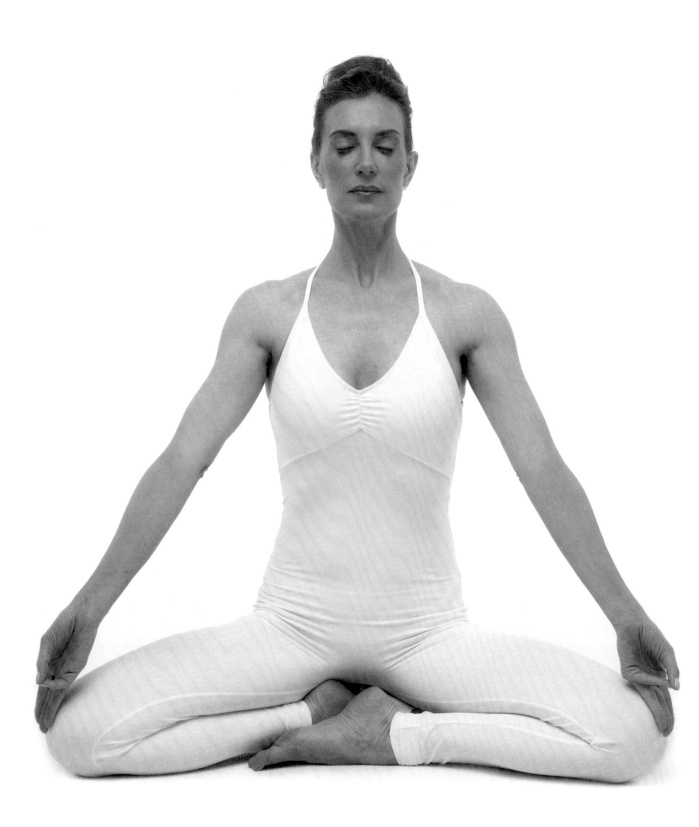

THE MIRACLE MANTRA

The mantra "Guru Guru Wahe Guru, Guru Ram Das Guru" (pronounced "*guh*-roo *guh*-roo *wah*-hay *guh*-roo, *guh*-roo *raam daas guh*-roo") means, "Divine teacher, servant of divinity which brings me from darkness into light, I am in ecstasy because of your greatness." It is known as the Miracle Mantra because of its seeming ability to generate miracles, which it does by aligning our soul with the love of the universe. The vibrational force of the Miracle Mantra elevates our radiance to the love frequency in a fast and profound manner. The mantra is transmuted from the heart into the energy field surrounding our physical body, creating an alignment of purpose to the infinite that clears blockages from the pathway into time forward and allows the flow of love to prevail. Once its vibration radiates into our aura, unaligned constrictions and limitations become neutralized. Our intention flows from our heart with great fluidity and ease. This mantra is known to bring so much healing and so many miracles that in the ashram community we regularly share stories of how this mantra cleared difficult situations with grace. It turns the inner potential into outer reality.

Guru
Guru
Wahe Guru
Guru Ram Das
Guru

THE MIRACLE MANTRA

1 Sit up with your spine straight. With your palms facing the sky and the tops of your hands resting on your lap, touch the thumb and pinky finger of each hand together. This mudra of communication will accentuate your connection with the highest frequencies of your being.

2 Begin to chant the words "Guru Guru Wahe Guru, Guru Ram Das Guru." As you chant these high-vibrational syllables, allow your voice to release out comfortably. Imagine the sound you are creating bathing every cell in your body with illumination. Think of your entire spine as an antenna sending waves of healing to the physical body and the electromagnetic space around you, your aura. You may even sense a feeling of a tangible mist after a few minutes.

3 Continue chanting for three to eleven minutes.

4 When you are finished, sit in stillness and observe the transformation.

○ MEDITATION FOR ECSTASY OF CONSCIOUSNESS

Wahe Guru

This meditation uses the mantra "Wahe Guru" (pronounced "*wah*-hay guh-*roo*"). A great workout, a yoga class, special time with someone we love, or a conversation we waited too long to have all elevate our state of consciousness. We call this "ecstasy." The following exercise can bring you directly into the ecstasy of consciousness.

1 Sit up tall with a straight spine. Rest your hands palms up on your knees, with the tip of each index finger and thumb touching in Gyan Mudra. Sit with gratitude and a feeling that you are filled with light, knowing you are valuable and being thankful for that truth.

2 Begin to chant, "*wah*-hay guh-*roo*, *wah*-hay guh-*roo*, *wah*-hay guh-*roo*, *wah*-hay guh-*roo*." As you chant aloud, imagine an activation occurring within you that removes all wounds and darkness. Reflect. Feel calm. There is so much to be thankful for. Believe it and receive it.

3 Continue chanting aloud for up to eleven minutes while you listen to the sound within and around you.

○ THE MUL (ROOT) MANTRA

One of the most powerful forces for change in kundalini yoga is the Mul Mantra, which means "root mantra." This mantra contains the root of sound that is the foundation of all mantras. It can uplift our frequency so that we attract exactly what our soul desires. Our soul longs for the very same things that God has planned for us to receive. While the mind may desire things on the basis of ego or personal, shortsighted gain, the soul desires only what supports our highest good.

When we operate from a vibration of fear, we attract more to be afraid of. But when we activate the high frequency of light that arrives every time we plug into God, we literally shift into a new potential. Our vibrational field speaks for us, and we attract that which we are.

When our desire, soul, and destiny are in all in alignment, the energy of the universe flows through us, but when our desire is self-serving and comes from ego, we cannot succeed. The Mul Mantra creates the proper alignment. The universe loves us, and we are meant to live lives that are happy and fulfilling. This mantra is one of the greatest tools for getting from point A to point B. It truly is that simple. This is a mantra we both chant continuously in our own lives.

The full mantra is this:

Ek Ong Kar, Sat Nam, Kartaa Purkh, Nirbhao, Nirvair, Akaal Moorat, Ajoonee, Saibhang, Gur Prasaad, Jap, Aad Sach, Jugaad Sach, Hai Bhee Sach, Nanak Hosee Bhee Sach

It is pronounced "Eck Ong-*Kaar*, Sutt-*Naam*, *Kar*-taa Poork, Neer-*baoh*, Neer-*vaire*, Uh-*kaal* Moort, Uh-*joo*-nee, Say-*bahng*, Goor pruh-*saad*, Jap, Aad Such, Joo-*gaad* Such, *Heh*-bee Such, *Naa*-nek *Ho*-see Bee Such"

We would like to share our personal translation of this mantra's meaning:

Ek Ong Kar "There is one infinite consciousness which creates all. Creator and the creation are one. As creation, I am one with the creator consciousness."

Sat Nam "Truth is universal identity. I am authentic, and my authenticity and truth are the gifts that God has given me." (When we chant "Sat Nam" we are affirming that truth is our identity. We are saying, "I am truth.")

Kartaa Purkh "God puts everything into action."

Ek Ong Kar

Sat Nam

Kartaa Purkh

Nirbhao

Nirvair

Akaal Moorat

Ajoonee

Saibhang

Gur Prasaad

Jap

Aad Sach

Jugaad Sach

Hai Bhee Sach

Nanak Hosee Bhee Sach

Nirbhao   "My true identity is without fear, exuberant and still at the same time. I am allowing the truth of divine identity to shine without concern."

Nirvair   "My true identity feels no anger or vengeance. I am nonreactive. I am responsible for my own situation and potential. I have the power within me to live my own truth, and if I am angry because I am not living my truth, it is simply time to reclaim my power."

Akaal Moorat   "My true identity is immortal. Beyond death. Infinite."

Ajoonee   "My true identity is not born, because it is timeless. I leave a legacy to the world by living in my truth."

Saibhang   "My true identity is perfect and complete. My spirit brings me everything I need, and this same energy can help others, too. My true identity is sparkling and healing to others."

Gur Prasaad   "Everything is a divine gift."

Jap   "Meditate on this, and meditate with focus, clarity, and positive intention, so that you can manifest all goodness forever and ever."

Aad Sach, Jugaad Sach, Hai Bhee Sach, Nanak Hosee Bhee Sach "Meditate on what was true in the beginning of time, throughout all time, now, and in the future. God is eternal and true."

EK ONG KAR SAT GURU PRASAD, SAT GURU PRASAD EK ONG KAR

Guru Prasad is the state of mind of total gratitude, the acknowledgment that all existence is a gift of the universe and is given to bring light to our consciousness. It is said that repeating the mantra "Ek Ong Kar Sat Guru Prasad, Sat Guru Prasad Ek Ong Kar" (pronounced "ekk onng *karr*, sutt gur-prah-*saad*, sutt gur-prah-*saad* ek ong *karr*") even five times can put the brakes on the mind when it is stuck in a thought pattern that is not serving you. This mantra is known to stop even thoughts that won't stop.

Ek Ong Kar
Sat Guru Prasad
Sat Guru Prasad
Ek Ong Kar

DEEP LISTENING

Whatever our souls are made of, his and mine are the same.
EMILY BRONTË

There is a silent sound in the universe. This sound is the perpetual vibration that connects us all with one another, our higher selves, and God. There is an infinite sound inside of us that fills our souls with comfort, ease, and the ability to surrender. This deep listening opens our sensitivity and intuition, and it is in this silence where we can experience the calmness the sounds create initially.

One of our greatest challenges in life is that we forget to listen. We actually forget there is sound when we cannot hear it with our two physical ears. We forget there is an inner ear that resides in the center of our hearts. This is the miraculous beauty of the unstruck sound. This sound is an internal vibration that will enable us to return to our natural state of love and unite body, mind, soul, and breath. When we close our eyes and listen deeply, we realize that we are part of a world of sound. Vibration is everywhere.

○ CONNECT WITH THE SOUND OF THE SOUL

If we are feeling fear or anger, the heart tends to shut down and the soul tends to hide under the rage of the ego. When our minds play games with us, it is the ego that comes out to play. These are times when we react to triggers, feeling the need to protect ourselves. Reacting from the standpoint of mind and ego is never beneficial and is never sustainable. The path of the soul is the path of truth, beauty, and love, which opens us to the abundance of the world. The path of the soul is the path of flowers, miracles, and beautiful gifts.

How do we get in touch with our soul? Beethoven said, "Music is the mediator between the life of the sense and the life of the spirit." The exercise of deep listening below creates a profound shift in consciousness that helps us recognize everything is exactly how it is meant to be. Everything unfolds in perfect timing. We recommend doing this seemingly simple but life-changing practice every day.

1 Sit comfortably and connect with the flow of your breath.

2 Close your eyes and begin to listen to the sounds around you. Do not listen to any one sound, but listen to the pure totality of sound, the way a baby would hear sounds without knowing what they are. Try to hear everything at once.

3 Allow them to enter your awareness and then release them without judgment. Do not get caught up in any one thought. All the thoughts you think have a sound, light, and vibration. Just observe. What are your thoughts?

4 Listen through only your right ear for a moment.

5 Listen through only your left ear for a moment.

6 Listen to the sounds inside the room for a few moments.

7 Listen to the sounds outside the room for a few moments.

8 Observe how the sounds change your energy frequency.

9 Keeping the eyes closed, observe if you see light in the midst of the sound.

10 To finish, whisper to your heart, "I love you. I care for you. Your sounds, words, and thoughts are beautiful. I do not need to react. I do not need to defend. I am enough with my gentle whispering of the heart."

Throughout the rest of the day, notice how frequently your mind begins to put you down. Recognize your insecurities are of the mind. When your mind starts to have thoughts that trigger you, say out loud: "There goes my brain doing that thing again." The negative thoughts are not real. They are simply grooved into the neurological network of the mind. Just as water always finds the lowest point in which to settle, your thoughts will trap themselves in that canal. However, you have everything you need within you right now to uplift and shift any stuck thought patterns. Fear is a choice, and love is another choice. While using the tools in this book, we invite you to make a commitment to choose love. Once love becomes your choice, you may observe your life changing in beautiful ways that more deeply express your inner truth.

PART 2

DIVING INTO KUNDALINI YOGA

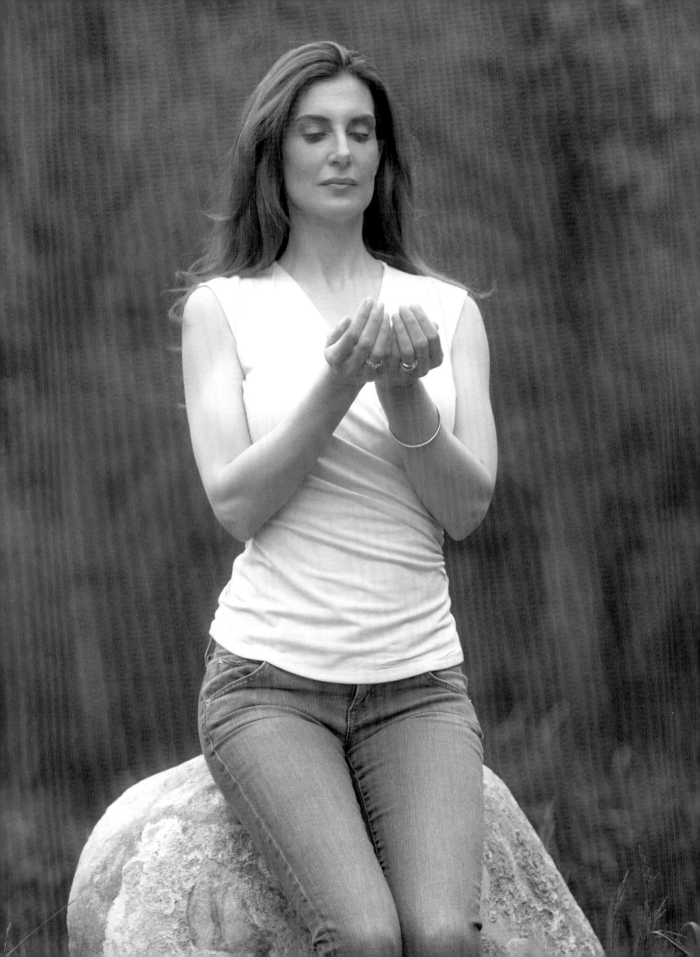

6 THIS PRACTICE IS FOR YOU

*You are already that which you want to be, and your refusal
to believe this is the only reason you do not see it.*
NEVILLE GODDARD

IN THE PREVIOUS CHAPTERS YOU heard about the keys that unlock
our energy and thinking with kundalini yoga. Now we will dive
deeper into the practice. In this chapter you will find key elements
of kundalini yoga that are especially helpful to know as you continue
your practice and start clearing your energy.

TUNING IN

Before we begin a yoga session, we first open an inner space of rev-
erence by bringing our awareness to our breathing, our body, the
prana that is flowing through all, and the sacredness in that prana.
We use a special mantra to vibrate and connect our inner self with
the creative infinite. Yoga opens us to the most sacred aspects of our

existence, the essence of our being, and the essence of all there is. As we open, we recognize that our individual consciousness and the divine grace of the universe are intertwined in never-ending and beautiful ways.

The following two practices are done to open the sacred space within our hearts prior to beginning a yoga session.

○ MINDFUL CENTERING

Instead of just diving into an exercise, it is important to first come back to our connection with our expanded nature. This is the stable platform from which we operate on the soul level. The practice called Nadi Sodhni is a way of tuning in with breath in order to clear our energy channels, be present, and open the inner space to the flow of your own energy. *Nadi Sodhni* literally means "to clear the energy channels of our body so prana can flow freely." The practice is simple but creates a dramatic internal change. Nadi Sodhni can be done before your yoga practice, but it is also a gift at any time to uplift your endeavors by bringing your entire being into alignment with the divine flow.

1 Sit up straight, close your eyes, and focus your attention on the third eye point.

2 Feel the aliveness of your spinal column as it aligns and rises up like a lotus stalk from your perineum to the top of your head. Sense the beautiful fragrance of your aura. Slow your breath down and observe the flow of love-infused prana entering your lungs. Visualize the prana the breath carries flowing through your spine, permeating every fiber of your body, and expanding into your aura.

3 Continue to slow your breath down, holding it in after the inhale and out after the exhale. Feel your presence in your body as one with the universe. Repeat for several breaths until you feel ready and aware enough to take on your practice.

○ ADI MANTRA

Repeating the Adi Mantra before we begin our yoga practice aligns our energy field with the creative energy of the universe. Just as the musicians in an orchestra will tune their instruments to a common note, this mantra tunes our being to the same frequency of consciousness as that of the lineage of spiritual teachers who have come before us.

Ong
Namo
Guru
Dev
Namo

The mantra is "Ong Namo Guru Dev Namo" (pronounced "ong nahm-*oh*- guh-*roo dayv*- nahm-*oh*"), and our translation is, "I honor the creative force of the universe, which is within me, around me, and beyond." *Ong* is the creative force of the infinite. *Namo* is the greeting of one divine essence honoring another, as light recognizing light. Combined together, "Ong Namo" is a mutual recognition and salutation in the realm of spirit between the finite creation of your own consciousness and the infinite creative force. *Guru Dev* means "the great enlightener," which is the force of the universe that brings us from darkness to light.

Repeat this mantra three or more times before any yoga practice. Take a moment after chanting to sit still while immersing yourself in the exquisite reverberation of the sound as pure soundless vibration.

1 Sit up with your spine straight. Close your eyes and press your palms firmly together in front of your heart with your thumbs against your sternum. Observe your breath flowing in and out through your nostrils, filling your lungs and abdomen while bringing light and love to your entire being. Imagine you are going to vibrate the words of the mantra into the totality of all creation and connect with the creative force behind it.

2 Take several deep breaths in and out through the nose.

Ong

Namo

Guru

Dev

Namo

3 When you are ready to chant, with the exhale, slowly form the sacred sound of this mantra: "Ong Namo Guru Dev Namo." Feel the vibration in your spine and third eye point. Envision the sound as it ripples into the space around and within you, in divine recognition of the creative force of the universe. The sound of the "o" wells up from the timeless depths of your abdomen and reverberates into the light channel of the spine and into the space around your body. The buzzy sound of "ngggg" resonates in the midbrain and at the crown of the head, opening the crown chakra to the wisdom of spirit.

4 Imagine the cord of light from the base of your spine to the crown of your head surrendering in devotion to the infinite creative force.

5 Repeat the mantra three or more times before you begin your yoga session.

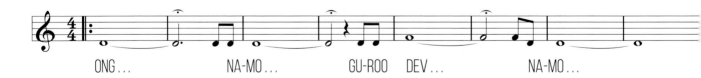

ONG...   NA-MO...   GU-ROO   DEV...   NA-MO...

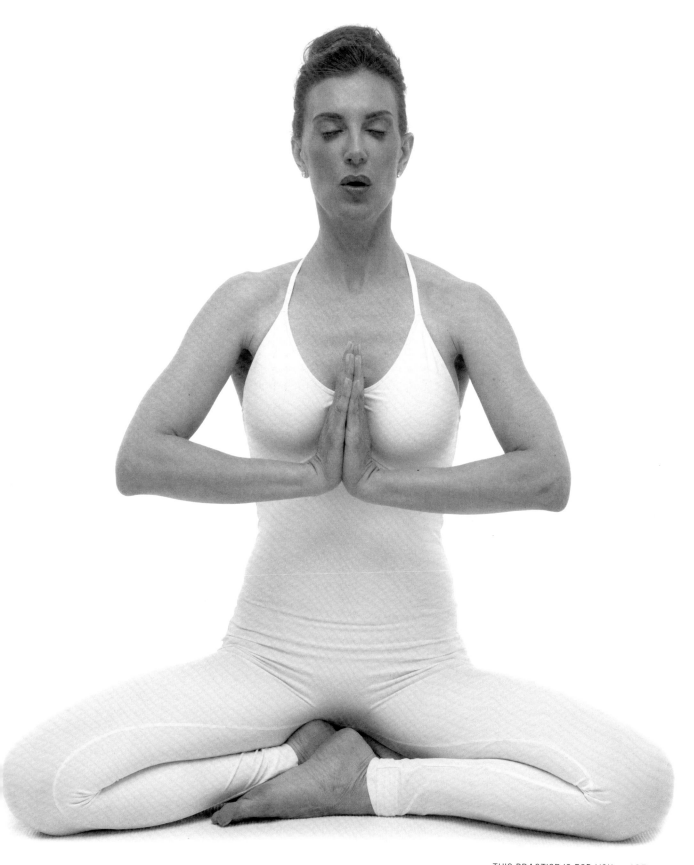

CLOSE YOUR EYES

Be still. . . . Stillness reveals the secrets of eternity.
LAO-TZU

One of the most beautiful aspects of practicing kundalini yoga is that we become aware of the subtleties within our body and the ripples of energy through our aura. These treasures of life are right inside us, and we can sense them with our eyes closed. Therefore, we practice most of kundalini yoga with our eyes shut. In life we spend so much time searching outside of ourselves for answers, yet the true wisdom can be discovered in still, inner silence.

At night we can see the stars in the dark sky, but in the day, there is so much ambient light we can't perceive them. Closing our eyes in yoga is like re-creating that night sky. We are able to become aware of subtleties that simply are impossible to see with the eyes open.

THIRD EYE POINT

The third eye point, the area between the eyebrows, is the natural resting point for our focus when we are not thinking about all sorts of other things. Concentrating on this point generates mental and emotional relaxation. It becomes the platform of repose for the mind, like a sacred altar. In the pages of this book, you will often come upon instructions to concentrate on the third eye point. This kind of attention is never tense. It's an easy, natural thing to do when we relax.

TIP OF THE NOSE

In many kundalini yoga exercises, we lower the eyelids nearly all the way down and gaze at the tip of the nose. This ancient practice quiets the mind and opens the sensitivity of the third eye. Normally our eyes are very reactive, reflexively looking in the direction of any motion that comes across the retina and also moving in response to our thoughts. For example, if you try to remember something from your childhood, your eyes will move as your mind searches for the memory. Even in our dreams the eyes roam around behind our eyelids in response to the images in our mind.

The optic nerve is a bundle of nerves that runs like a highway through the center of our brain; it has a major branch going to the pineal gland. The pineal gland in turn influences our melatonin production, our sense of calm, and our sensitivity to subtle shifts in the electromagnetic field. By lowering your eyelids, drawing your eyes inward, and looking at the tip of your nose, you will allow the more sensitive impressions reaching the third eye to be discerned and your mind to quiet itself. This is a scientifically based physiological response. By doing this, we stabilize the optic nerve impulses that trigger the motor neurons creating eye movement.

If your mind is racing, try this technique. As you hold your gaze at the tip of your nose, observe your mind beginning to slow down.

STEADY PRACTICE

Steady, patient practice makes for steady progress. Having a rhythm to your routine—whether it is every day, every other day, or three days a week—creates a frequency, and a frequency creates a vibration, and a vibration can move mountains. We have found that if you practice every day, or at least three times per week, you will see amazing progress. Life begins to flow. Doors begin to open. There really are not words to describe the magic. The only way to experience it is to do it.

Ideally, try to practice in the early morning before dawn, the traditional time to do kundalini yoga. The hormonal changes that occur naturally in the quiet predawn hours make our bodies receptive to the deep energy shifts that start developing with kundalini yoga practice.

CREATING SACRED SPACE

Your vision will become clear only when you can look into your own heart. Who looks outside, dreams; who looks inside, awakens.
CARL JUNG

We have the ability to create a sacred environment so that our homes become a space of safety and comfort, a reminder to be disciplined in our practice and our self-care, and a place to create a routine in our lives that connects us to our higher selves. Our home can reflect back to us our inherent divinity and grace. Set up a space for your practice that is clear of distractions, technology, and clutter of any sort. On a small table, we can make an altar with pictures and objects that connect us to spirit. Anything that speaks to our highest consciousness and helps us feel uplifted can be placed on the altar.

Creating sacred space often requires the removal of other objects that clutter our field of consciousness or that carry a negative emotional charge. Clutter is a huge energetic distraction in our lives. Everything holds energy, and anything that is not loved, needed, or valuable can be given away. When we release objects rather than holding on to them, we open space for new love and energy to enter our lives. This is the concept of *prana and apana*. Until what we need to eliminate energetically, apana, is released, prana will be restricted. Recycling is a form of giving back, and the universe always returns the favor. Less is more. Let go of what you do not need or love, so more beauty can enter your field.

MOVING THROUGH ENERGETIC BLOCKS

Keep up and you will be kept up.
YOGI BHAJAN

You may find yourself feeling frustrated at times as your newfound energy starts to seem impeded by walls of long-held resistance. As we are doing an exercise, we often find ourselves before an inner wall where our mind will start fabricating all sorts of reasons to stop. The breakthroughs happen when we stay with it—but not to the point of injury. When you feel like giving up, consciously breathe and ask yourself, "Is it my mind, or is it my body?" This is a crucial distinction. We have to discern between our mind's unhealthy resistance and our body's healthy warning signs. We have seen people trying to power through their pain, which is a dangerous course to take whether in daily life or in yoga. It is important to cultivate inner sensitivity to our body. Be aware of your intuition, your inner dimension, and your physical condition and forgive yourself if you are not where you want to be. Life is not a race, and you are exactly where you are supposed to be. Kundalini yoga is noncompetitive and noncomparative. Wisdom and sensitivity carry the day. If we always follow our heart wisdom rather than the expectations of the mind, we will find the balance we need to keep steady in the face of challenge.

Once we determine that the blocks of the mind are causing the resistance, we can choose to stay with the exercise and continue breathing deeply. We will often then notice that we have moved past our self-imposed wall and into a beautiful new inner vista. Always and invariably, however, another wall will come up. Whether one is a beginner or a longtime master, the inner work is exactly the same. There are infinite walls and infinite breakthroughs and infinitely more beautiful vistas. The process is one of addressing each new challenge that feels tailor-made to meet us where we are.

By concentrating in a relaxed yet focused way, we can often continue beyond what we thought were our limitations. Moving past our limits is not about creating tension or fighting something. It is about softening, breathing, and filling yourself with so much light that your awareness dissolves into it. With regular practice our body and mind gain the capacity to stay steady, relaxed, still, and centered, even in the face of challenge.

YOUR MIND IS NOT YOU

God and Mind, and Mind and God are not two things.
One is the vehicle, and one is the destination.
YOGI BHAJAN

As we clarify our awareness with kundalini yoga, we start to see our own mind more clearly. Our mind is one of the most remarkable machines, constantly sorting, analyzing, inventing solutions, creating categories, making sense. We love our mind. But we are not our mind. The mind is a powerful steam engine, yet it needs an engineer to drive it. The engineer is you—the soul that is coupled to your heart.

A mind without a boss is like a runaway train. It keeps shoveling coal into its own fire and chugging down a track—even when it's the wrong track. The mind actually isn't all that smart. It is the locomotive engine whirring away at lightning speed and coming up with ideas every millisecond. But it needs our soul to say when it is right or wrong.

In ancient India they called it the "monkey mind," because it jumps around like an untrained monkey from thought to thought without focus. One day we feel loved and adored, and the very next day we wonder why we said what we said and if we might have upset someone and whether what we did will cause everything to come crashing down like a line of dominoes. On a Saturday we feel like we have things figured out, and by Wednesday we worry we are making every mistake possible. These are the illusions the machinery of the mind creates.

The lens that the mind tries to see through is often distorted by false perceptions or vibrations from past traumas caught in the subconscious and echoing in the aura. The mind creates false scenarios based on past experiences, and these influence the present moment.

Our work in our yoga practice is to train the mind to sit still, see clearly, and be ready for action when we need it. We develop a volume knob, a tone control, and an on-off switch. Then our mind becomes a fabulously useful gift—a servant rather than a tyrant.

Once we start trusting our heart to direct our path, the mind will follow by figuring out how to implement our soul's callings on earth. This is when synchronicity begins to unfold.

Did you know that scientists discovered the heart has a brain of its own? The heart of a fetus begins beating before the brain is even developed. The heart has a neuronal complex with billions of synaptic connections. The brain of the heart knows that love rules everything. Trusting the heart over the mind can make us feel frightened and vulnerable. However, learning to trust this inherent wisdom of the heart is one of the greatest powers of the kundalini yoga practice.

When we soften inward, we are melting into the arms of the divine and allowing soul-level direction. Most of us were not brought up to understand that the soul is in the driver's seat or that the mind can be a tool to serve our soul's mission. Love, kindness, and upliftment are our soul-level quests, the opposite of overthinking, contracting, and reacting.

THE PROBLEM WITH THINKING

Where there is love, there is nothing impossible.
YOGI BHAJAN

It is practically impossible to alter our thought patterns by thinking. In the self-help world we are sometimes advised to choose good thoughts in order to be healthy and whole, but the reality is that thinking our way out of established patterns is an unattainable goal. Although we feel called by a force in our soul to allow our energetic beauty to shine, it's like climbing an ice mountain. Our first impulse is to hold on with a white-knuckled grip to an outdated mental map book that actually no longer serves us. We try to do the "right thing," even though underneath we may feel it isn't. Often we have practiced patterns of thoughts that undermine our fulfillment all our lives. These patterns become powerfully ingrained vibrations persistently distracting our attention. Think as we may that we would like to change, we easily slide back and find ourselves enmeshed in old patterns, spinning the same thoughts, and going to sleep with the same old fears that we know are not good for us. We can feel powerless to get free of this cycle, and the feeling of powerlessness itself can become an even steeper slope of ice that keeps us sliding and spinning. So what do we do?

What we have found is that by releasing physical tension you can release the thought patterns that hold that tension in place. The physical work of kundalini yoga allows your soul-level energy to clear the whirlpools of energetic vibration that thinking creates. As you practice the exercises on the following pages, you may find that you can perceive your mind with a new perspective. You can start to see the pattern of thinking as different from you. As you feel your kundalini energy become activated, it grows so much brighter than the whirlpools of thoughts. The clear, quiet, persistent voice of our soul keeps becoming stronger. This is a fascinating process, and no one can say for sure how it works. However, when the soul leads through the heart, those old, habitual patterns of thinking seem to dissolve in the brilliance of your own light.

NATURALLY SPIRITUAL

Make friends with the angels, who though invisible are always with you. Often invoke them, constantly praise them, and make good use of their help and assistance in all your temporal and spiritual affairs.
SAINT FRANCIS DE SALES

Human beings are naturally spiritual. The feeling of connection to a force greater than oneself is one of the most compelling drives common to all of humanity and throughout all of history. The impulse to align with what we feel as a mystical, spiritual power calls us to action the same way our drives for food, shelter, and sexuality do. The feeling of spirit is inherently a personal experience.

In kundalini yoga we welcome the experience of spirit. It happens! We do not preach. We allow. We find that when we break through the blockages of our energy and our prana begins to flow, a natural, heightened sense of our own divinity often breaks through as well. When we relate to our spirit, we allow our purest energetic potential to flow through our being. We open the door to the angelic dimension, and this is where divine guidance can come through.

Many emotions well up in kundalini yoga as we meditate and move our energy. People have a profound deepening of awareness and clarifying of vision. Often this leads to tangible and direct spiritual experiences. It is so common to feel deeply in the practice of opening that we almost take the tears flowing in a kundalini class as a normal occurrence. They are tears of release and tears of remembering who we are. It is a natural part of being truly human. It is the washing away of energetic clutter. It is the bliss that comes from a catharsis.

TIMING YOUR PRACTICE

Yesterday is gone. Tomorrow has not yet come.
We have only today. Let us begin.
MOTHER TERESA

Presetting a specific amount of time for each exercise creates an intention that can help you transcend what you thought your limit was. If you are new to kundalini yoga, take it easy on your body and listen to what your intuition is saying about how long to practice. It is fine to practice an exercise for less time than specified in the instructions and often fine to go longer, too, but whatever length of time you choose, we encourage you to set the intention to finish so you receive the sense of fulfillment that comes with completion. As you progress, you can gradually increase the amount of time you practice.

Throughout this book, we have suggested a range of times for the practice of each exercise, designed to address from beginning- to advanced-level practitioners. We leave it to you to determine what works best for you.

ENDING YOUR YOGA SESSION

The final inhalation at the end of a yoga, chanting, or meditation practice is a powerful moment of integration. The cessation of movement doesn't mean the exercise is over. It means the door has been opened, and now is the moment to step through it. Give yourself time to truly assimilate the shifts in your energy, hormones, and blood flow before you run off to do something else. Stay seated and conscious for at least a minute and preferably longer. It is during this quiet time that we often reach new realizations. We have seen so many people just jump up from the mat as soon as their last position is over and miss out on a crucial part of the process. Please give yourself this gift of time to be aware. It truly is the moment you have waited for. And then carry it with you into your day, your steps, and your words. In a kundalini yoga class, the session is traditionally finished with a sweet song and three repetitions of the mantra Sat Nam to contain the energy that has been generated.

We like to think of this moment when we end the practice as the receiving of a gift. It is similar to the pause between the inhale and the exhale. It is the moment we stop doing and we begin being. This is the space where miracles happen. It is the moment of still perfection that attracts light and love with ease. Hold on to the feeling of this moment and practice coming back to it all day long. In this way the yoga session never really ends.

RELAX

The human expansion from individual self to
universal self is through the art of relaxation.
YOGI BHAJAN

When our body relaxes instead of constricts, we open ourselves to the love-infused prana that is always available and coursing through us. Like ocean waves at the beach, waves of energy in the earth's magnetic field wash away the havoc and hassles of the day, leaving us shiny, bright, pure, and alive. Our entire being integrates—mind, body, breath, soul, aura, and radiance. We reconnect with the most subtle and important aspects of life that otherwise go unnoticed in our whirlwind of daily activities.

Rather than working toward changing anything, we simply allow ourselves the pure delight of surrender. We relax into the arms of the divine. The parasympathetic nervous system takes charge, and our body rebalances internally. True healing occurs, starting in our very core.

○ DEEP RELAXATION

The most fundamentally important pose in all of yoga is deep, conscious relaxation while lying on the back. A yoga session typically ends with a practice of Deep Relaxation three to thirty minutes long. But you do not have to have done any previous exercise in order to do this one. Simply lying down for eleven minutes at any time during your day and following the instructions below can change your entire outlook. During this period of nondoing, a great deal goes on internally. It is when the most dramatic shifts can occur, if we allow them to.

In Deep Relaxation we can completely let go. We begin to see with new eyes that everything is perfect just as it is. A golden thread of divine order runs through our lives. We see that everything we experience is here to help us grow into our best version of ourselves. We are reminded of the short life we are given, and we are offered an opportunity to awaken into our highest potential by evolving, trusting, and allowing the universe to do its work.

Our circulation can relax as well, so covering yourself with a shawl or blanket will help you keep from getting chilly. Find a firm but comfortable mat or carpet to lie on. Our natural receptivity to visible light affects our hormones, even when light hits anywhere on our skin, so keep the lights switched off or as low as possible, especially those that might shine directly into your third eye point.

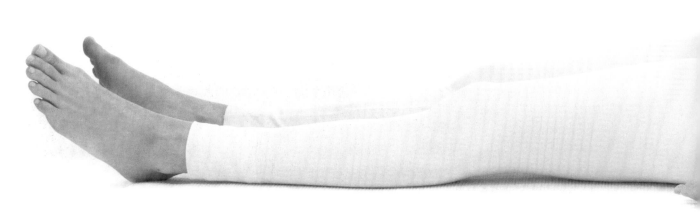

1 Lie down onto your back and cover yourself with a light blanket or shawl. Place your arms alongside your body with your palms facing the sky and legs spread at least shoulder width apart.

2 Allow the weight of your legs to surrender to gravity, your feet to let go of the need to move, and your toes to open out toward the sides. Surrender as though you could not even think of moving. Melt your limbs, torso, and head into the ground and feel the loving presence of the earth supporting and encouraging you.

3 Slow down your breathing, feeling the flow of breath through your nose and up past your third eye. Feel your breath as light and love flowing deeply into your body, and feel that light flowing through the electromagnetic field around you.

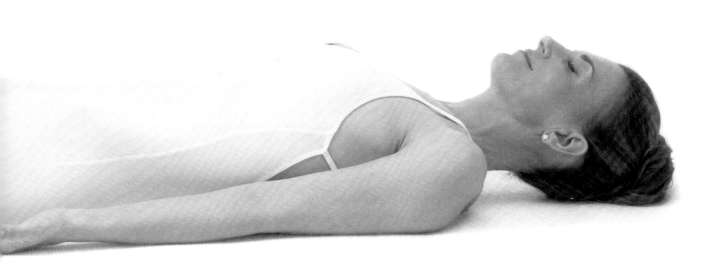

4 Feel the energy of the universe as interwoven with your own energy field, washing through your aura and clearing away blocks. Feel grace and love washing away tension and cleansing areas of resistance in your energy field. Allow yourself to heal. Receiving is your birthright. This is a magical moment. Trust that you are enough; trust that you are loved.

5 Continue for three to thirty-one minutes.

6 To return from Deep Relaxation, first bring your body back to conscious movement by rotating your wrists and ankles. Then briskly rub the soles of your feet and your palms together, stimulating the nerve endings and reinvigorating your circulation. Hug your knees to your chest and rock forward and backward on your back several times to reset your magnetic field. Then sit up and feel refreshed, brightened, and connected.

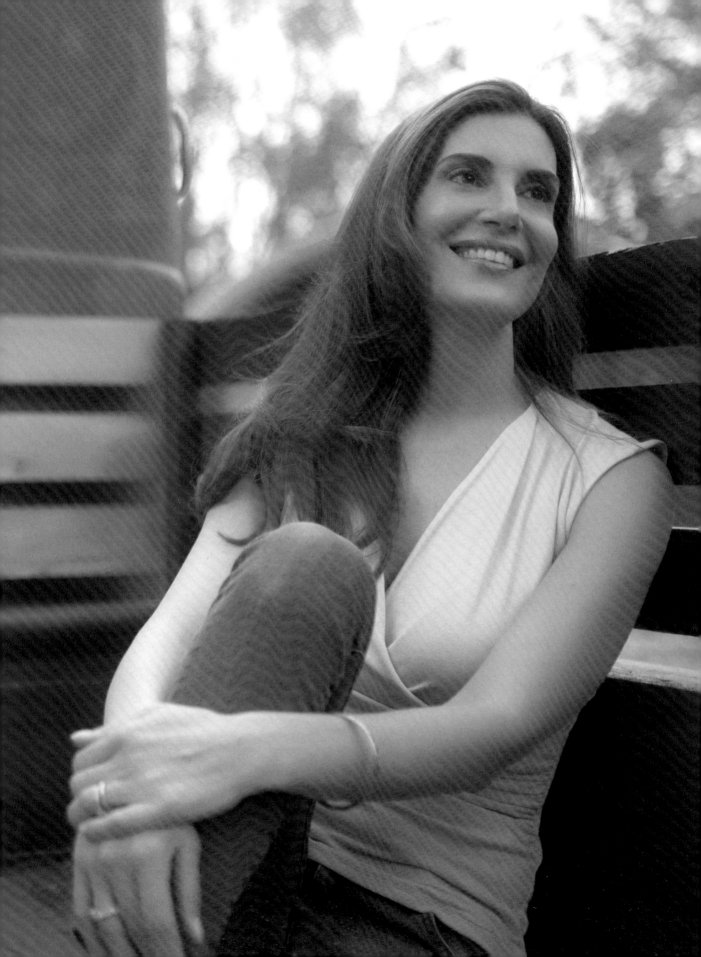

7 ESSENTIALS OF KUNDALINI YOGA

Your task is not to seek for Love, but merely to seek and find
all the barriers within yourself that you have built against it.
A COURSE IN MIRACLES

WE HAVE CHOSEN TO GO into depth with the following selection of kundalini yoga techniques because of their ability to move our pranic energy through our body and electromagnetic field so transformation can occur. These are basics that will support your journey to open your heart and allow your soul to shine. Practicing them will provide a tangible experience of how changing our energy alters our body and how using our body shifts our energy. You will find many of these exercises again and again in the traditional kundalini yoga sequences that are discussed later in the book.

○ **BHANDAS** ENERGY LOCKS

Bhandas, also known as *energy locks*, are core practices of kundalini yoga. They awaken, unlock, and unite the flow of our bioenergy through the central channel of the spine. They stimulate the kundalini and direct its flow through a clear, open pathway of the *shushmuna*, the energy pathway along the spinal column. Bhandas combine suspending the breath with a subtle tightening of specific muscles so as to move prana through our energy pathways, activating our higher centers of awareness.

The pranic energy they work with is quite sacred, which is why the locks have sometimes been surrounded by an air of mysticism. These locks were held secret for thousands of years because they instill an incredible potency. This power is not something to be afraid of—it is a power to be claimed. Your soul is ready to reclaim the devotion for itself that you may have given away for most of your adult life, and your heart knows this. We cannot urge you enough to practice using bhandas to awaken your inner shine.

The three main bhandas are Root Lock, Diaphragm Lock, and Neck Lock. Below we have described them as individual yoga practices in order for you to learn them. The locks are often applied during the final breath of a kundalini yoga exercise. However, you can practice the locks in any position at any time: sitting, lying down, and even (more lightly) while walking.

A note about pronunciation: we give the classic names for the locks as we describe them below, but in the rest of this book we stick with the English names to make these practices more accessible and user-friendly. Our intention is to welcome you to the experience (rather than the language) of the practice.

◯ ROOT LOCK

Root Lock activates kundalini energy at the base of the spine, awakening the boundless energetic potential of our true self. Sexual energy is the limited way that much of the world experiences this power, and most of us are familiar with how compelling sexual energy is. But there is much more to this energy than sexual arousal. Once you learn how to make it flow, it becomes the reservoir of your entire life-force.

Root Lock is called *Mul Bhand* (pronounced "*mool* bond") in the original language of India. Root Lock is most often practiced while suspending the breath—either in or out—but can also be done for a period of time while breathing fully. A light Mul Bhand is held during most kundalini yoga exercises. It can also be practiced at any time—in your office, while walking, or going about your day.

1 To learn Mul Bhand, sit in an upright position and feel your spine rising from your pelvis to the top of your head. Connect with the flow of prana through your nostrils and into your being.

2 Exhale all your breath out, fully emptying your lungs. Hold it out while you contract the muscles of the perineal area: tighten the area around the anus and perineum and draw the sex organs up and back toward the lowermost vertebrae. Draw the bellybutton back toward the spine. Visualize the concentrated energy within the entire pelvic region being directed to the base of the spine. Continue to hold your breath out and apply the lock for as long you can. Embrace the freedom of letting your energy activate your diamond brilliance.

3 When you feel ready, release the muscles and slowly inhale, visualizing your breath as light that interacts with your soul. Sit for some time as you transition into breathing normally, allowing your prana to circulate to every cell of your body.

4 You may wish to repeat Root Lock one or two more times.

○ DIAPHRAGM LOCK

In the area of the solar plexus, the life-force prana mixes with the eliminative force apana. One can't flow without the other, but once we connect them, our deepest energy can move unimpeded through the spinal pathway. Without Diaphragm Lock, our kundalini has a hard time rising from the base of the spine to the level of the heart. Diaphragm Lock opens the door to this energetic pathway, allowing our prana to flow up past the diaphragm so our heart becomes touched, illumined, and resonant with the light of our soul.

Diaphragm Lock was traditionally called *Uddiyana Bhand* (pronounced "oo-dee-*yah*-nah bond"), which means "to lift up." You can think of Diaphragm Lock as an energetic and anatomical platform for the heart. The base of the heart is in fact supported with tendons that attach it to the diaphragm. As we touched upon earlier, when the heart has a grounded and strong platform to rest upon, it feels safe to open. Diaphragm Lock gives us this beautiful means by which we can live through our hearts with grace.

The awakening of the heart is deeply profound and absolutely essential on the journey of our consciousness. The short pathway of kundalini energy from the navel to the heart generates a true breakthrough in consciousness. It requires letting go of a sense of self, safety, and security and trusting that our heart can carry us with light and love. Once our prana enters into the realm of the heart, our life source surges. We become connected with all those around us. It is as though the heavens open in us and our energy can flow in ways it was prevented from before. Also, when the heart is open, the mind quiets. When the mind stills, the heart can be the boss. When the heart is in charge, our lives become magical playgrounds full of fun and loving synchronicity and moments of perfect bliss.

1 Sit up with your spine straight in a space conducive to honoring your own spirit.

2 When you feel ready, exhale entirely and lift the diaphragm up toward the heart. This will draw the navel in, pulling

it back toward the spinal column. Remember, the diaphragm is like a stiff trampoline that can be lifted up toward the heart or pushed down toward the navel.

3   Feel the unimpeded flow of light rising through the channel of energy in the center of your spine. Prana that was blocked and held in the lower chakras can now flow unimpeded from the base of the spine into the rib cage. Let it touch your heart so it can blossom like a beautiful flower made of light.

4   When you feel ready, very slowly and consciously release the lock and inhale again. You may wish to repeat the lock two or more times.

○ NECK LOCK

The third bhanda, Neck Lock, allows prana to move up through the neck, awakening the third eye and pituitary gland and radiating into our aura. Neck Lock opens the fifth chakra—the throat—so kundalini energy can flow to the sixth, seventh, and eighth chakras. Without Neck Lock our energy is often blocked at the throat, and our soul light cannot reach the higher chakra frequencies of intuition, sacred wisdom, and surrender to the divine. The traditional yogic word for Neck Lock is *Jalandhara Bhand* (pronounced "jahl-unn-*dah*-rah bond"), which literally means "neck lock."

Sometimes we experience a sense of fear when we begin to connect deeply to spirit, and we pull back from the cosmic breakthrough that happens when energy flow reaches the third eye and awakens intuition. If you feel fear, please remember that prana is love. There is no reason to do any of this except to awaken and blossom so the fragrance of your soul can be sensed as part of you. The third eye is where we discern the unseen reality behind the surface, the eternal ebb and flow of the energy of life. The intuition requires complete neutrality in order not to shrink back. The crown chakra, at the top of the head, is the gateway to our rare divine consciousness. And in the aura we become an integrated, coherent whole rather than a series of separate chakras. The line between our finite idenity and infinite consciousness becomes blurred. We blend. We are not separate.

1 To practice Neck Lock, first make sure you are in a conducive space. Take a moment to connect with your breathing while seated or standing.

2 Draw the chin back and slightly down while lifting the back of the head and stretching open the spaces between the vertebrae in the back of the neck. Allow your chest to rise and ribs to expand, keeping the shoulders relaxed. This will straighten the curvature at the back of the neck. It is a gentle tug rather than a forceful position, and it should be held anytime one is sitting, during meditation or breathing exercises as well.

3 Take a moment to feel the flow of energy rising to awaken the third eye, the crown chakra, and your aura. Breathe long, deep inhales and exhales.

○ MAHA BHAND

When the three locks—Root Lock, Diphragm Lock, and Neck Lock—are practiced all together at once, as they often are, we call it Great Lock, or *Maha Bhand* (pronounced "*mah*-hah bond"). Maha Bhand enables the totality of our energy to flow as one unimpeded circuit. We vibrate as a coherent energetic flow of love, our soul identity. In general, you can always choose to practice the Maha Bhand at the finish of a kundalini yoga exercise for one to three breaths.

○ SAT KRIYA

Sat Kriya (pronounced "sutt kree-yah") is a single phenomenal exercise that imparts all the benefits of kundalini yoga; it has the power of many other exercises in one. It is a deep healing practice that balances all aspects of the self. Perhaps the most famous exercise in all of kundalini yoga, Sat Kriya offers a superquick fix for moving, balancing, and stimulating the energy along the spine while enabling it to be assimilated with the electromagnetic field. This energy integration can happen in as little as three minutes with Sat Kriya. We love this exercise, and we have suggested it to thousands of people who have claimed it gave them new life experiences.

Sat Kriya opens the flow of prana to rise through the central channel of the spine and opens the shutters of the crown chakra at the top of the head, allowing our consciousness to blend with the loving grace of the infinite. Sat Kriya connects the flow of kundalini by merging prana and apana at the level of the diaphragm. Sexual energy merges into accessible vitality and creative force as it rises from the second chakra, filling the energy channels all the way up our body while enhancing our radiance around the body. Overall, Sat Kriya develops our ability to stay centered, focused, and at the same time expansive. If you have time for nothing else, practice Sat Kriya for three minutes in the morning and watch how your day goes. It is absolutely life changing to practice Sat Kriya for three to thirty-one minutes daily.

Sat Kriya combines three things: a body position, a repetitive motion at the navel point, and a sacred mantra, "Sat Nam," which is described in depth in chapter 5. When doing this exercise, give yourself sufficient time to relax afterward, and do it in a place where you will not be disturbed and you can chant out loud without any fear.

Sat Nam

1 Sit on your heels on the floor and breathe deeply. Feel the flow of prana coming in through your nose as you fill your lungs. Radiate love energy throughout your body as you exhale.

2 Draw the chin back slightly so your neck is in Neck Lock. Extend your arms straight up overhead with the elbows alongside your ears. Put your palms together and interlace your fingers, keeping only the index fingers stretched straight up and pressed together. Feel the elongation extending from the base of your spine all the way up to your fingertips, as if your fingertips were drawing light up from your root chakra.

3 Throughout the exercise, simply allow your breath to come and go as feels natural. It typically sneaks in as a little sniff after the "Sat" on its own. It's best not to pay much attention to your breathing in Sat Kriya and allow it to happen automatically.

4 Draw the navel in sharply toward the spine while continuing to extend the arms and hands up and powerfully say the mantra "Sat" out loud. Then release the navel and say the mantra "Nam" out loud. Repeat, drawing the navel in on each "Sat" and releasing it on each "Nam," creating a steady rhythm slightly slower than one per second. Continue for three to thirty-one minutes.

5 To finish, inhale as deeply as possible. Apply Root Lock and focus on your third eye point. Visualizing it as a bright white light, draw your energy up the spine, through the top of the head, and up to the fingertips. Hold the position while suspending your breath for ten seconds.

6 Then exhale all the breath out as you release the lock and visualize the energy flowing out through the top of your head.

7 When you have fully emptied the lungs, repeat Maha Bhand while holding the breath out for ten seconds. With the breath held out, the navel can be drawn back farther into the abdomen. Imagine light rising up from the base of your spine to your fingertips. Again, exhale completely and picture the light surrounding your body.

8 Repeat the inhale and exhale two more times, maintaining Maha Bhand as you hold the breath after the inhalation, for ten seconds each time. Then, with full awareness, slowly and gently bring your arms down and transition to normal breathing.

9 Lie down on your back and allow the flow of energy to do its magic. Just relax every fiber of your body. Take long and deep inhales and long and complete exhales. The energy flowing has its own wisdom. Trust that everything is as it needs to be in this moment. Continue to relax for at least as long as you practiced the exercise, if not longer.

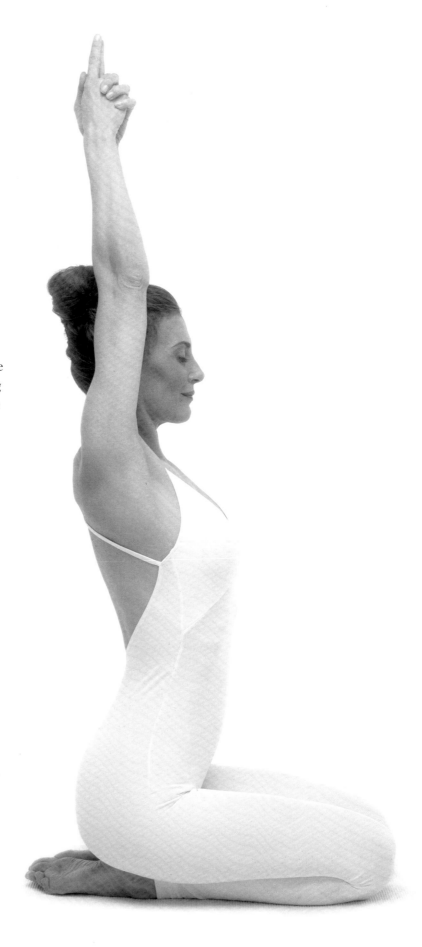

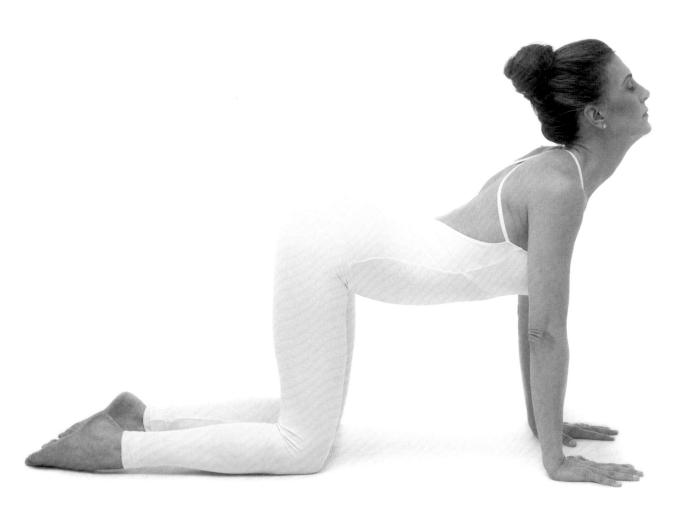

○ CAT-COW

Cat-Cow keeps your spine flexible and your heart open while integrating all of your chakras. The fluid back-and-forth movement of the entire spine, from coccyx to head, promotes the exchange of cerebrospinal fluid and allows us to experience the flow of life. The steady tipping motion adjusts the hormone-producing glands, in particular the thyroid, increasing the metabolism, helping with weight loss, and energizing us for our entire day. The spinal fluid moves up to the brain, releasing the feel-good neurotransmitters and bringing a vitality to our thinking.

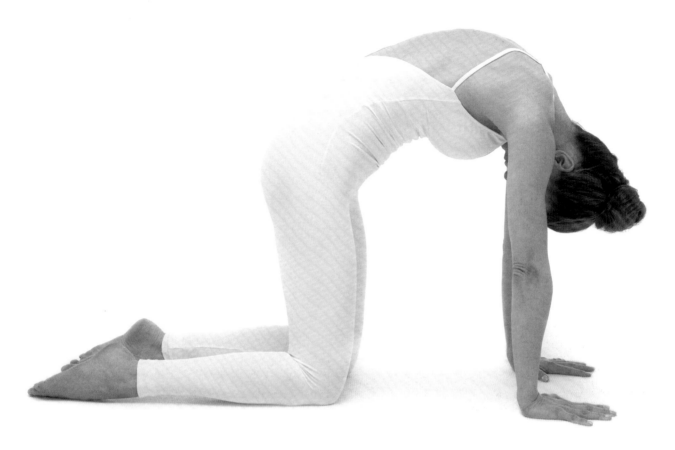

1 Come onto your hands and knees on the floor, with your knees directly under your hips and your wrists directly below your shoulders. Feel the stability of the pose as you root yourself to the earth on all fours.

2 Inhale as you open your heart toward the sky, lifting the chin and expanding your rib cage. Explore the space between the vertebrae and see if you can move one vertebra at a time when you begin to stretch your spine. Notice where you are flexible and where you feel stiff.

3 Exhale as you press your hands into the earth and round the spine upward like a Halloween cat, tucking the chin in toward your chest and the tailbone in toward your navel. Again, try to move one vertebra at a time.

4 Continue this movement for one to three minutes. Once you feel you have warmed up, you may speed up, but be careful never to whip the neck up and down. Always stay present and focused on your inhale and exhale so that the breath leads the movement. The breath moves the spine, and the spine moves the rest of the body.

5 To finish, inhale deeply in the up position, hold your breath, and apply Root Lock. Hold for five to fifteen seconds, then release.

○ ADVANCED CAT-COW WITH KNEE BEND

This is a great exercise for keeping the glutes toned while stimulating the powerful immune system of the spine. It also balances the neurotransmitters, bringing clear freshness to the mind. The extension of the leg behind the body works the muscles in the back and gives the spine a nice adjustment.

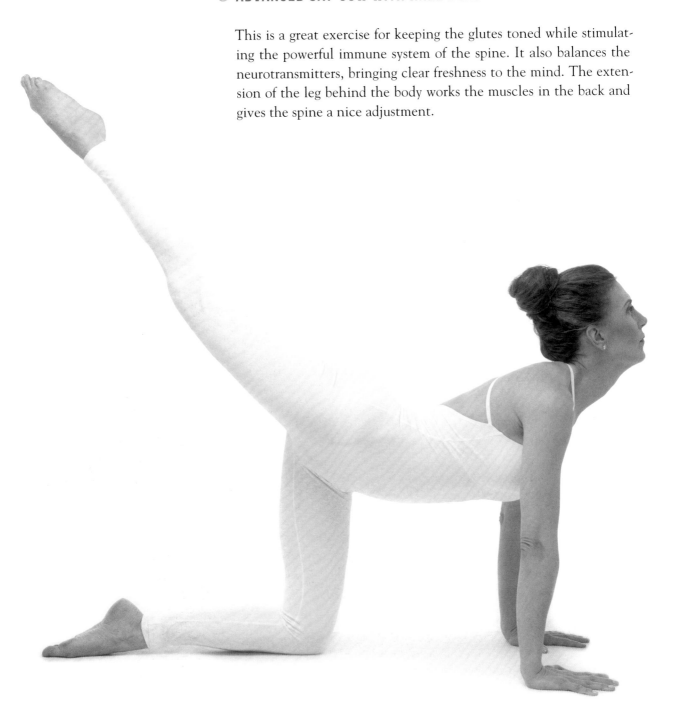

1 Begin in the same position as in the regular Cat-Cow, as described above.

2 As you inhale, extend the left leg high behind you, straightening the knee. Open your heart toward the sky, lift the chin, and expand your rib cage.

3 As you exhale, round the back, lower your head, and bring the left knee forward so that you are almost touching your forehead with your knee.

4 Repeat steps 2 and 3, continuing for one to three minutes. Then switch sides and do the exercise for an equal length of time on the opposite side.

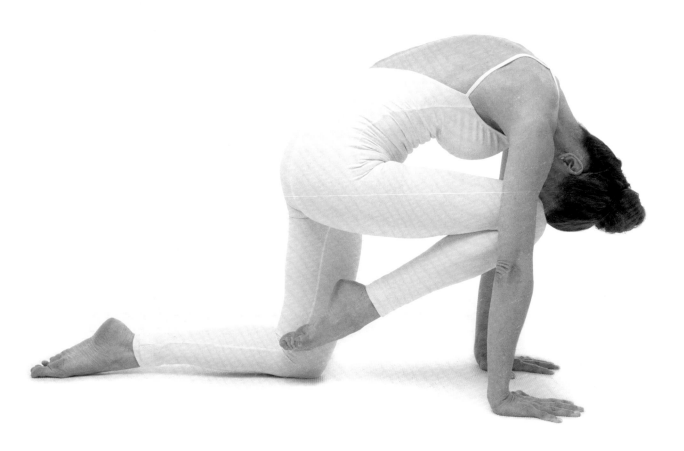

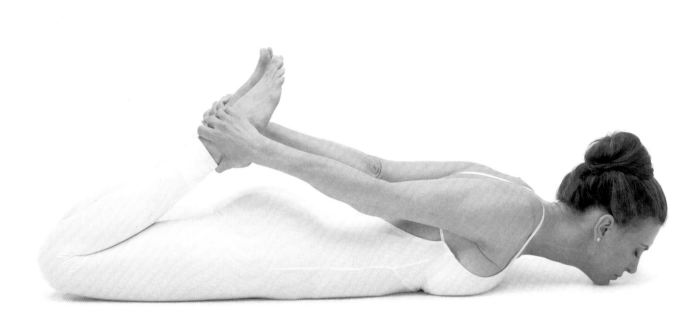

○ BOW POSE

Bow Pose opens the heart energy of the fourth chakra and allows it to rise up to the sixth, seventh, and eighth chakras. It releases constrictions in the lungs and thyroid, which increases our metabolism and internal fire and can promote weight loss and boost energy all day long. This pose stretches the abdomen wonderfully, releasing trapped prana that may be causing constipation and menstrual cramps. It relieves a great deal of lower back tension. Bow pose is used in many kundalini sets and is an excellent pose to practice on its own.

1 Lie down on your stomach. Bend your knees, reach back with your hands, and take hold of your ankles. Take several long, deep breaths as you stretch the fronts of your thighs by pulling on the ankles.

2 While holding on to your ankles, inhale, arch your back, raise your chin, and lift everything you possibly can up off the floor and toward the sky. Deepen your breathing and feel how the inhalation increases the stretch. Continue breathing long, deep breaths for thirty seconds to three minutes while holding the position. Alternatively, you may practice Breath of Fire while in this pose.

3 To finish, while still holding your ankles, inhale deeply, arch up fully, and then exhale completely. Apply the Root Lock with your breath held out. Inhale and repeat a second time.

4 To come out of the position, slowly inhale as you relax your body down. Once your knees are on the floor, release the ankles from your hands and rest on your belly, resting on your cheek with your head turned to one side. Take your time and simply allow the opening of energy flow along the central nerve channel of your spine.

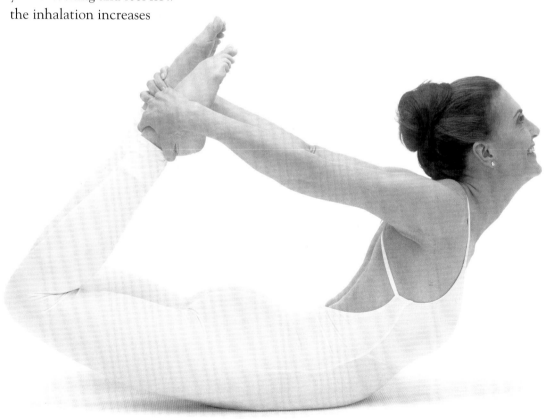

○ FROG POSE

If you want an exercise that tones your glutes and thighs while at the same time moves pranic energy through the spine and deepens your breathing, Frog Pose is for you! As we move the pelvis and lower spine through the electromagnetic field and stretch the hamstrings, we release blockages in the flow of prana through the fronts and backs of the thighs and through the first and second chakras. This pose is so beneficial. It gives you a spring in your step, self-confidence, and creative energy. It increases the flow of energy through the spine and even helps prevent cellulite. The back-and-forth tipping of the cranium works on the connectivity between your pituitary and pineal glands, and the motion stimulates the flow of cerebrospinal fluid, bringing freshness and clarity to the mind. If you have issues in your second chakra, like difficulty with fertility or hormonal imbalances, focus on pressing your heels together with intensity during the exercise; there are meridian points in the heels that stimulate energy in the second chakra.

Frog Pose is often done vigorously and rapidly, but it is fine to move and breathe slowly, holding and deepening into the positions. Being present, moving consciously, and making sure your breath is orchestrating your movement are the most important things to focus on.

1 Squat down onto the balls of your feet, with your heels pressed together and lifted above the ground. Press the tips of your fingers onto the ground in front of you, straightening your elbows and spreading your knees to either side of your arms. Lift your chin and expand your ribs, raising your heart up toward the sky.

2 Inhale, lift your hips, straighten your legs, and let the top of your head come straight down toward the ground. Keep your neck and lower spine relaxed and your heels touching together off the floor.

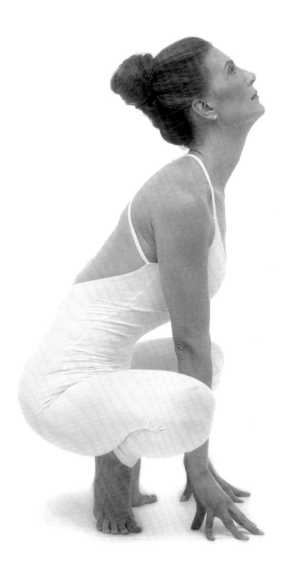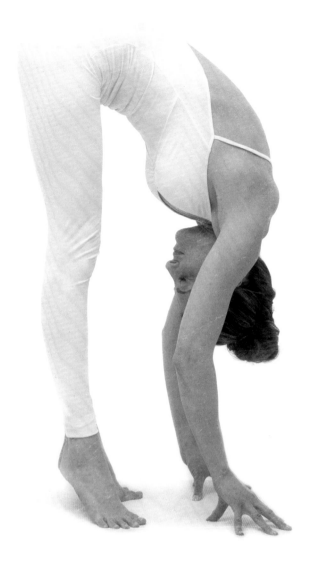

3 Exhale and return to the squatting position as in step 1, lifting the head so you are facing directly forward and raising the heart upward again.

4 Continue for twenty-five more lifts at your own pace.

5 To finish, lift the hips, hold the breath, and hold the position to consolidate the energy. Then exhale completely while relaxing down to the starting position.

○ BABY POSE

Relaxing in Baby Pose with the head lower than the heart creates a sense of wonder and lets the mind surrender to the wisdom of the fourth chakra. The head is tipped forward, energizing the third eye and the intuition, stimulating the pituitary and pineal glands, and opening us to activation of the self. In yogic terms this pose was called "the tipping of the cup of nectar so the moonbeams could be caught," because it permits the fire of the solar plexus to rise. Allow yourself to deepen into Baby Pose, slowing the breath down. Allow and surrender.

This is a wonderfully soothing exercise for children. Rubbing a child's lower back while they are in this position is very healing. Softly humming or chanting a mantra while nurturing them in this manner is a lovely way to comfort a loved one.

1 Sit on your heels and bring your forehead down to the ground or, if the floor is hard to reach, to a folded blanket in front of you.

2 Rest your arms alongside your body, with the palms face up next to the hips. Feel a separation between the shoulder blades as you give in to the force of gravity.

3 Breathe deeply and feel how as you inhale you gently open the space between your ribs and vertebrae. Relax into the pose and hold for as long as you feel comfortable.

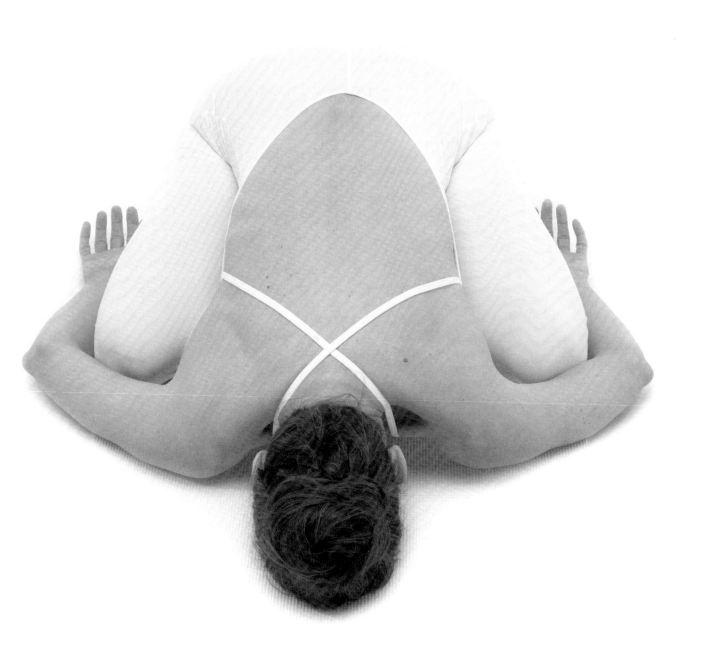

○ AURA CHARGER

As described in chapter 2, the eighth chakra is the dynamic electro-magnetic field around the body, called the aura. Illnesses are often stored as energetic blockages in this field before they even enter the physical body. We also hold imprints of childhood trauma in this energy field as well as imprints from our ancestors and their life experiences. It is essential to keep this field purified. Just as we take a shower to clean the physical body, we can use practices from kundalini yoga to cleanse our energy field.

Our absolutely favorite exercise for the eighth chakra is Aura Charger. This meditation can cleanse away toxic densities from our energy fields in just a few minutes. It combines Breath of Fire (as described in chapter 4) and a sixty-degree arm position to make your aura clear and let your radiance shine into the world.

1 Sit on your heels, keeping your spine straight and tall. Feel your breath entering your lungs and expanding your ribs. Close your eyes, bring your breath under conscious control, and observe the flow of prana past your third eye point with each inhalation and exhalation.

2 Curl your fingers so that your fingertips touch the pads on the palms just below each finger. Extend your thumbs away from your palms.

3 Stretch your arms up from your shoulders at a diagonal, as if you're pulling a rope between your hands, so they form a sixty-degree angle between them. Straighten your arms and keep your elbows locked, elongating the distance from your heart to your thumb tips.

4 Holding this position, do Breath of Fire for thirty seconds to three minutes. As you perform Breath of Fire, become aware of a line of energy flowing from your heart up through your shoulders and arms and into your fingertips. Feel this energy extend as an arc of brilliant light curving overhead from thumb to thumb and charging your aura with loving goodness. This arc will clear your aura of debris and energy blocks. Keep your shoulders relaxed and down so your heart is as open and filled with light as possible.

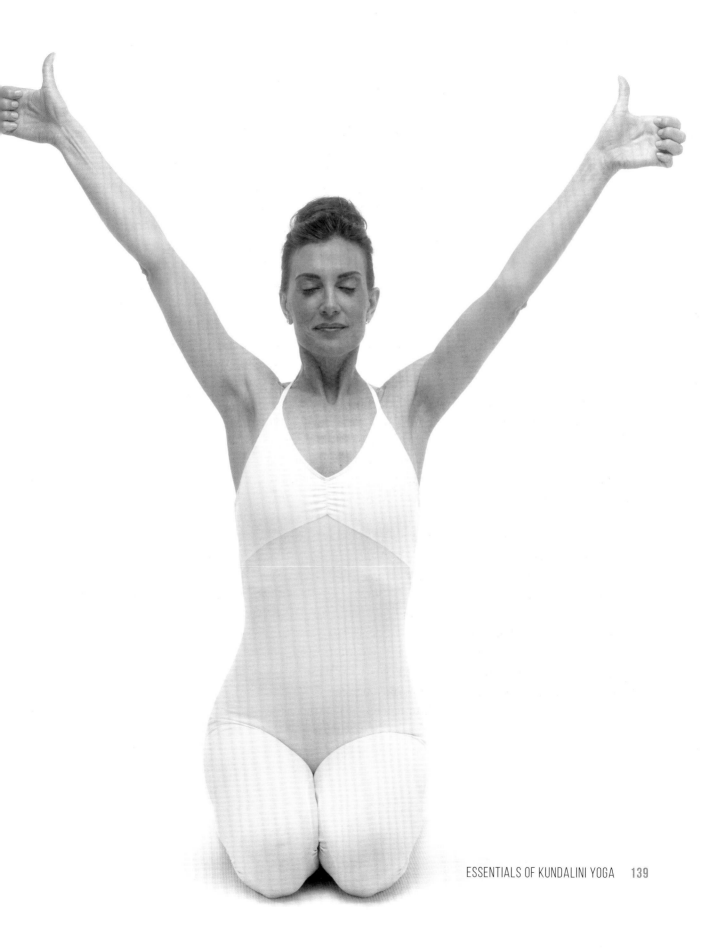

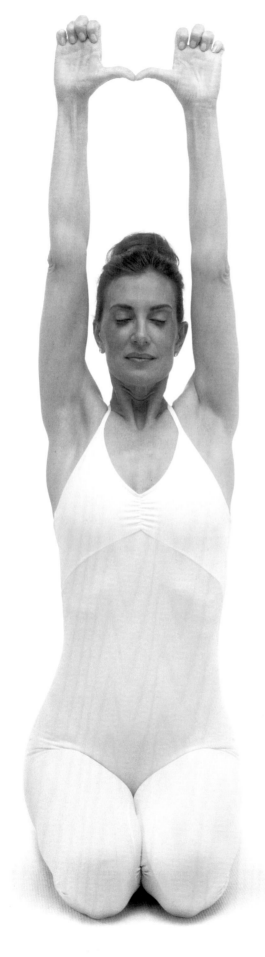

5 To finish, inhale deeply while stretching your arms straight up overhead and pressing the tips of your thumbs together. Suspend your breath, apply Root Lock, and stretch your spine up from your pelvis, opening the spaces between your vertebrae.

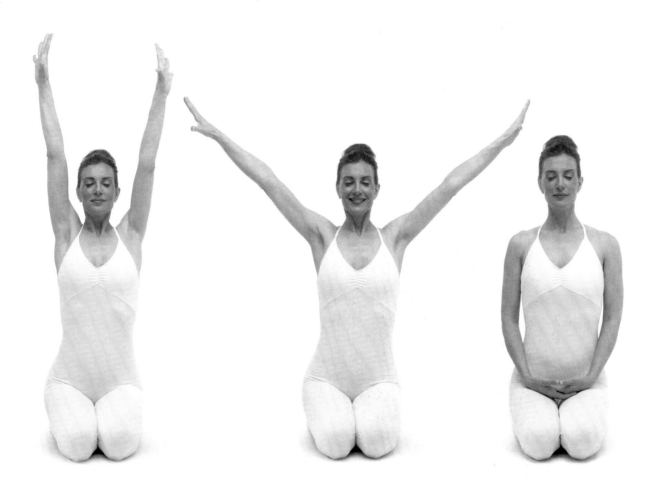

6 Exhale, extend your fingers with the palms down, and sweep your arms out and around you. We invite you to visualize light coming out of your fingertips to seal any rips in your energy field around your heart. Comb through your aura with your fingers, removing toxicity, negativity, and disease. As you clear the negative energy with your hands, imagine you are releasing it down into the earth below you. You are purifying the darkness from your aura, illuminating it with a bright white light.

7 To close, lower your hands onto your thighs with palms facing upward. Feel your energy circulating up from your spine, into the arc line above your head, and out into your aura. Visualize the pure and beautiful light you have created. Give yourself the precious gift of sitting, breathing, and being aware of the changes in your aura for as long as you can. Tune in to the energy that is you. It is love.

○ POWER ARCHER

Power Archer is the stance of the spiritual warrior. Think of your-self as strong but open to the divine. Wise but full of grace. Steady but willing to surrender to the flow of the universe's intelligence. Power Archer says we honor that everything is in divine order, and at the same time we are strong and are willing to stand for what we believe in. If you have difficulty concentrating, staying with an endeavor, or seeing the details, Power Archer can benefit you. It can also help you activate a dream and allow your infinite potential to manifest into reality.

Power Archer releases blocked energy in the lungs and heart, and it stimulates the thymus gland. It tones the muscles of and opens the hips while sending pranic energy into the lower vertebrae. The stretch in the pelvis frees the current of life-force so that we flow in synchronous dedication to the energy of the universe.

1 Stand up tall, feeling your spine rise elegantly from your hips. Breathe deeply into your abdomen and allow your shoulders to relax. Tune in to the sensation of weight distributed evenly between both feet. Feel your body elongate, rising against gravity from your feet to the top of your head.

2 Lunge a few feet forward onto your left leg so your knee is bent directly over the foot. Keep the right leg straight behind you and your weight evenly distributed between both feet so that you feel a balanced stretch across your pelvis. Turn your right foot a bit shy of ninety degrees.

3 Extend your left arm out straight in front of you, as if you were holding a bow. With your right arm, draw an imaginary arrow back, pulling your right elbow backward and parallel to the ground.

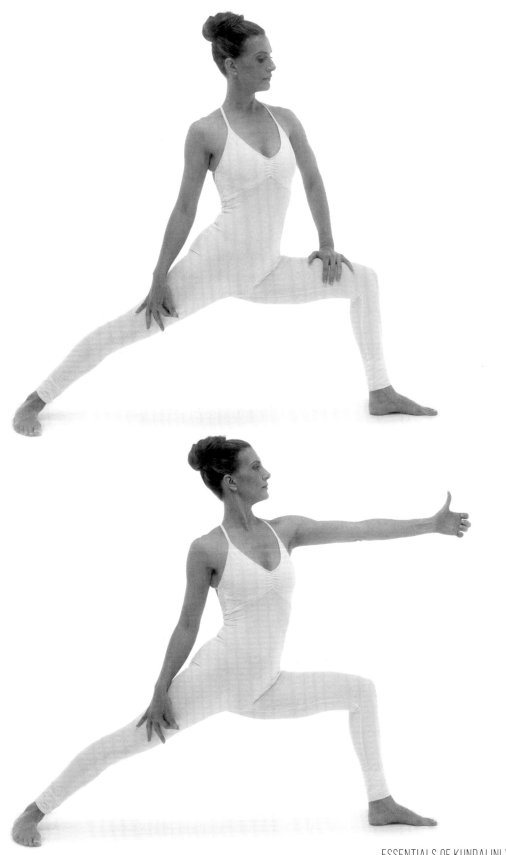

4 Widen the pull between your right elbow and the left hand, opening up across the ribs while keeping a lift in the right elbow. Make your spine long, tall, open, perpendicular to the earth, and flowing, like a light tube of energy.

That arrow you are aiming is the arrow of your intention. As you hold the pose, keep your eyes open on your target and imagine you are keenly training your arrow on your greatest dream. You are seeing it right in front of you and visualizing it as clearly as possible.

5 Begin Breath of Fire while holding the pose steadily and powerfully. Continue Breath of Fire for one to three minutes.

6 Inhale profoundly into the depths of your abdomen, aim your arrow, and let it fly as you release the breath. We invite you to feel the flow of energy from the earth below you. Feel your strength and your ease at the same time. Remember you are grace, but you are not a doormat. There is a huge difference between being soft, vulnerable, open, and spiritual and being a victim of an attack. This exercise is a great way to merge your power with your grace so that they go hand in hand.

7 Repeat steps 2 through 6 on the other side for the same length of time.

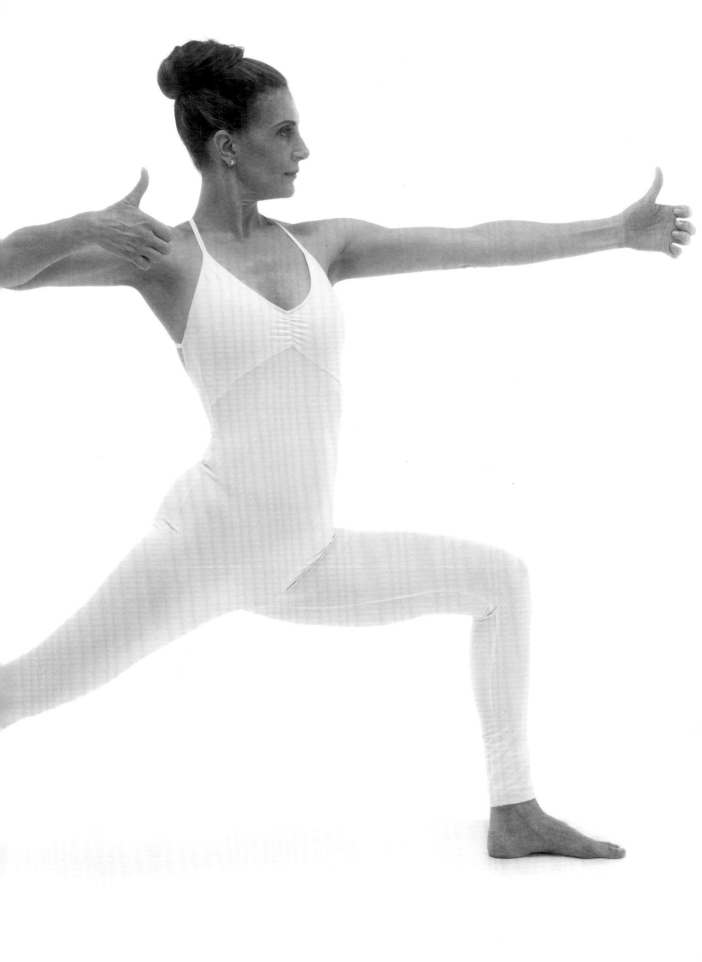

○ FLOW AND GLOW

Flow and Glow fills you with sparkle and luminescence. It gives clarity and freshness to your energy and your mind. Flow and Glow is a classic exercise. It is great to practice during flu season to boost the immune system. Flow and Glow keeps cerebrospinal fluid fresh and free of toxins. The undulating spine movement in Flow and Glow accelerates the circulation and recharging of the cerebrospinal fluid like a wave. It clears energy blockages in the spine and sushmana.

Flow and Glow is one fluid movement that flows seamlessly with the breath. Throughout the movement, lead with your chin and let your spine follow. As with most kundalini yoga exercises, coordinate your breath with the movement by exhaling as you arch your back up and compress the ribs and then inhaling as you drop the belly down and expand the rib cage.

1 Sit upright on your heels with your palms or fingers touching the ground on either side of your legs and your spine elongated. Connect with the breath flowing deeply in and out of your abdomen and the lovely energy flowing from the base of your spine to the top of your head.

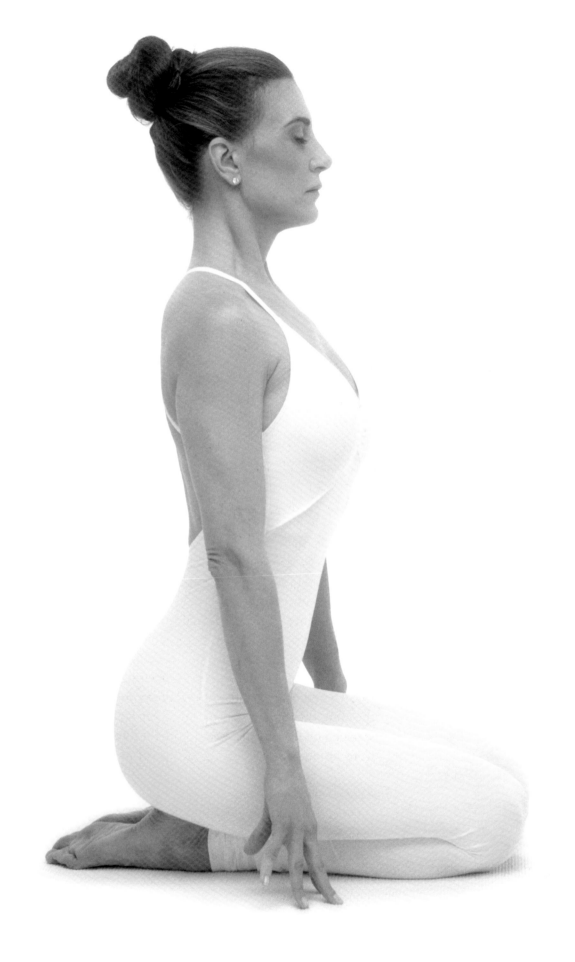

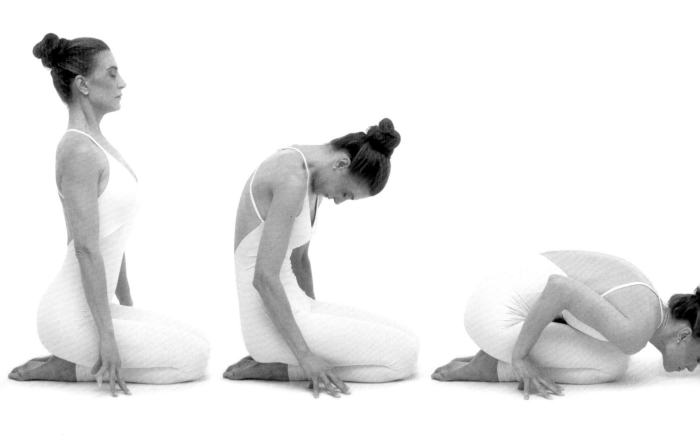

2 Leading with your chin,
exhale as you begin to
lean forward, bending your
elbows, bringing your
chin forward and down
toward your chest, and
allowing your spine
to curve forward.

3 Continue bending forward
so that your chin comes
down as low as possible,
either to the ground in
front of your knees or as

close to the floor as you
can bend. Arch your back
and bring your torso onto
or as close to your thighs as
you can. Feel the force of
gravity pulling you down.

4 As you inhale, begin to
lift your torso back up in a
smooth motion. First lift
the chin; then bring your
spine up off of your knees.
Keep lifting until you are

sitting tall, with your lower
spine flexed fully forward.

5 Repeat steps 3 and 4,
continuing the motion for
three minutes or longer.
Come down on the exhale
and up on the inhale,
creating an undulating
movement with the spine.
Keep your awareness on the
light flowing through your
spine. It is love. It is healing
you. It wants your success.

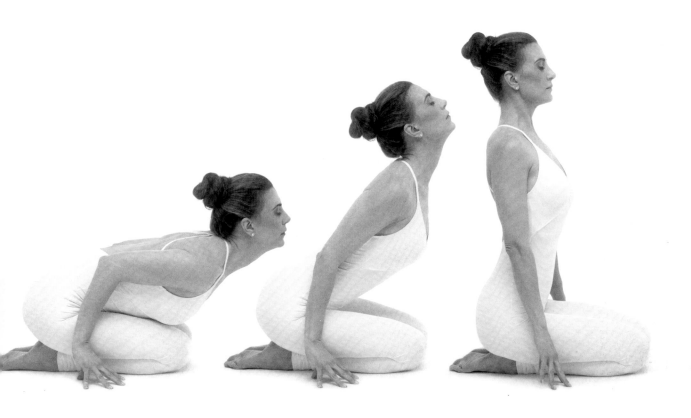

6 Sit up very straight and inhale deeply. Hold your breath in and perform Root Lock, drawing the perineum, rectum, sex organs, and abdomen up and in, awakening prana from your lower energy centers. Hold Root Lock with a steady, firm, supportive pressure, but without applying tension. Feel your energy awaken, flowing into the base of the sushmana and rising like a beautiful luminescence through your spine, activating your chakras, reaching to the top of your head, and radiating into your aura. Feel yourself being blessed.

7 Exhale and repeat Root Lock with the breath out.

8 To finish, inhale deeply into your abdomen; then exhale completely. Breathe normally with long, slow, steady breaths. Lie down onto your back, turn your palms upward, and relax completely. Don't try to control a thing. Let the energy of the universe flow through you, washing away disease and tension. Surrender.

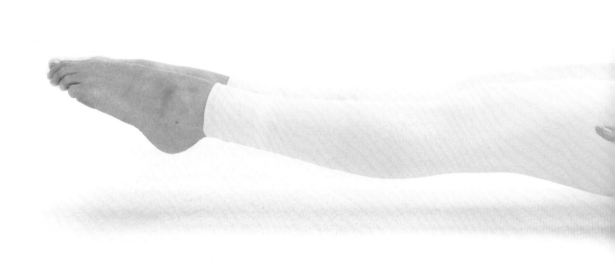

○ STRETCH POSE

Stretch Pose is a challenging posture, bringing sharp focus and presence to the body and mind in a very short time. On a physical level it tones the core muscles of the both abdomen and lower back, helps with digestion, and balances the adrenaline- and insulin-producing glands of the pancreas.

Strengthening the navel center fosters a sense of security in the natural connection between your spiritual self and your physical embodiment. When your core is strong, you have a platform from which your heart can feel safe opening. When the abdominal area is weak you will feel an emotional need to close off the heart in order to provide a false sense of safety. Living through the heart with vulnerability is the calling of this time. Yet if we are not strong in our navel, we will be too afraid to listen to our heart songs. Being a spiritual warrior means knowing that you are a powerful person who owns the gift of peace. Always remember that your grace is your biggest power.

Do not be afraid if your body begins to shake during Stretch Pose. The shaking is simply a sign that your nervous system is rebalancing.

It is quite normal to feel emotional after Stretch Pose. The emotions are being released, and that release is a blessing. Channel the energy you are experiencing into a fire that burns through any pain, physical or emotional. If you feel angry at the end, do the pose all over again and purge the frustration through the practice.

Please do not practice Stretch Pose if you are pregnant.

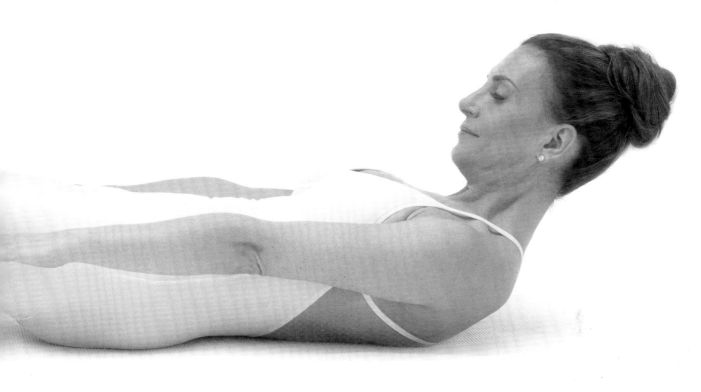

1 Lie down on your back. Recognize a cord of energy from the top of your head to the tips of your toes, with your navel at the center of it.

2 Tuck your chin toward your chest and lift your head, hands, and heels six inches off the ground. The neck and shoulders come up, but the rest of the back, including the shoulder blades, remains pressed into the ground. Straighten your fingers and stretch your arms out powerfully from your shoulders, with your elbows straight and parallel to the ground. Point your toes.

3 Begin Breath of Fire. Tune in to the current of invigorating energy from the top of the head to the tips of your toes. Continue for fifteen seconds or longer, building up to one to three minutes over time.

4 Inhale deeply, hold the position, suspend your breath, and focus your energy at your navel center. Exhale consciously while lowering your head and arms down.

5 To finish, simply lie still on your back, allowing your body to assimilate the effects of the pose. Breathe consciously and relax. You have just energized seventy-two thousand nerve endings at your core while releasing tension that was stored in your muscles and in your electromagnetic field. You may even feel a bit of a catharsis. Just surrender and allow it as part of your expansion of consciousness.

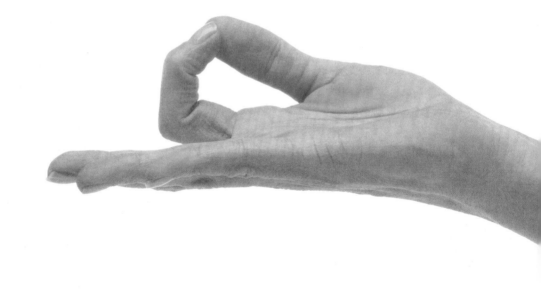

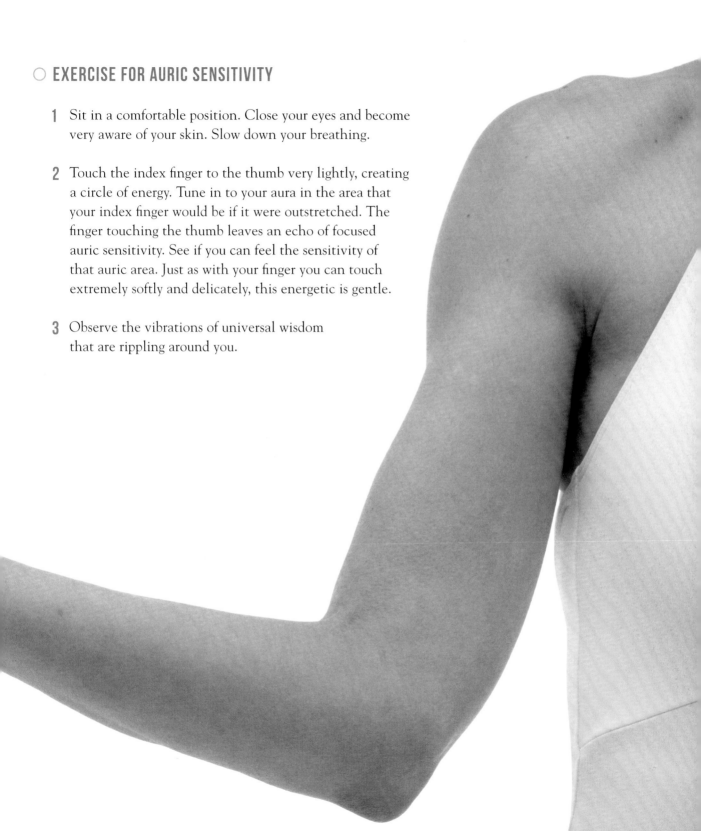

○ EXERCISE FOR AURIC SENSITIVITY

1   Sit in a comfortable position. Close your eyes and become very aware of your skin. Slow down your breathing.

2   Touch the index finger to the thumb very lightly, creating a circle of energy. Tune in to your aura in the area that your index finger would be if it were outstretched. The finger touching the thumb leaves an echo of focused auric sensitivity. See if you can feel the sensitivity of that auric area. Just as with your finger you can touch extremely softly and delicately, this energetic is gentle.

3   Observe the vibrations of universal wisdom that are rippling around you.

PRAYER POSE

Bringing our palms together in the center line of the body balances the left and right hemispheres of our nervous system, thereby balancing our focus. The millions of nerve endings in the palms and fingertips communicate with one another when our palms touch. When the many distractions of life are pulling you away from the grace of your own concentration, simply joining the palms together can recenter and rebalance your energy, bring you back into the present, and remind you of the timeless patience of your soul.

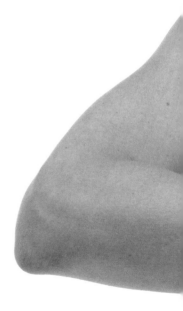

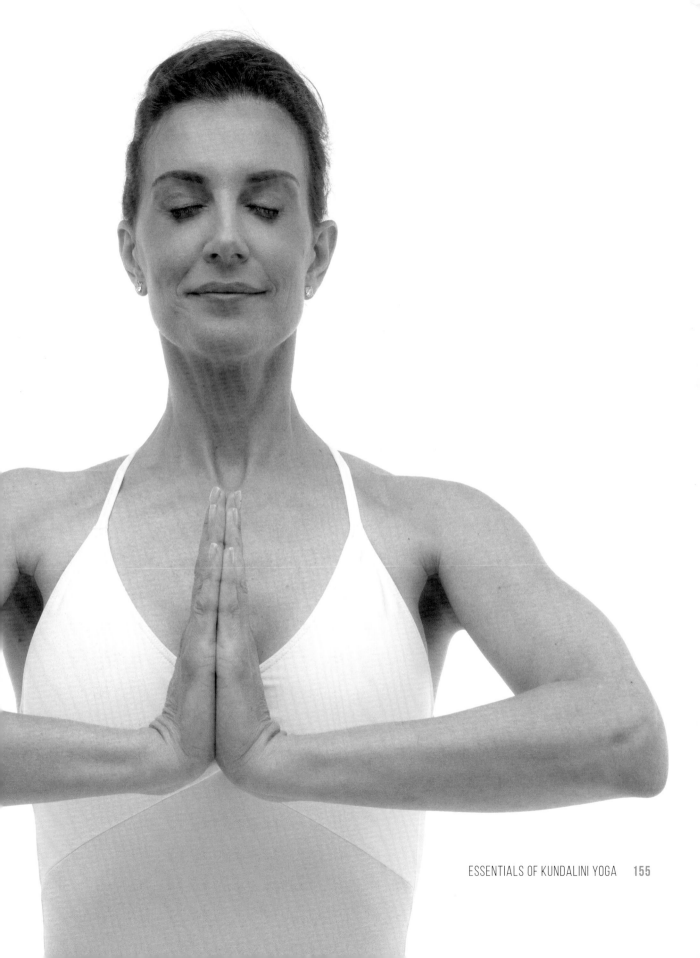

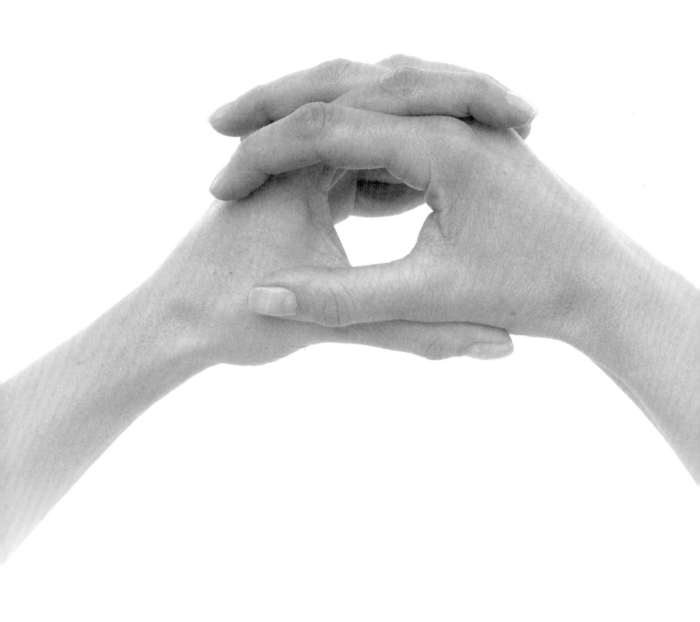

VENUS LOCK

This mudra channels sexual energy and helps balance the glands. Where the thumb connects into the palm is a raised mound called the Mound of Venus. The goddess Venus is the representative of beauty, grace, sensuality, and sexuality. The thumb represents the ego, or the falsely empowered identity of self as separate from the soul.

To do Venus Lock, fold your hands together, interlacing your fingers and resting one thumb on the Mound of Venus of the opposite hand. Traditionally, women place the thumb of their left hand upon the Mound of Venus of the right hand; for men, the right thumb rests on the left-hand Mound of Venus. It is a very balancing mudra that is often used in kundalini yoga exercises. You also can do it at any time during your day to generate vitality and a calm, knowing focus.

STRETCHING IN KUNDALINI YOGA

You surrender to a lot of things which are not worthy
of you. I wish you would surrender to your radiance,
your integrity, your beautiful human grace.
YOGI BHAJAN

Stretching the physical body is similar to the lifestyle philosophy shared throughout this book. Stretching is not about pushing or struggling. It is the gentle art of persistence that takes us from point A to point B. Pushing and struggling to get somewhere send messages to the universe that we do not trust our dreams will appear with grace.

Breath is the key to stretching in kundalini yoga. Breathe into a stretch by breathing fully into the depths of the abdomen. Embrace the feel of a stretch rather than retracting from it. Tightness in any area of the body is due to the restricted flow of prana, which in turn is caused by self-limiting beliefs or other stuck thinking. By breathing fully, we release the trapped prana. As the prana gives up its resistance to movement, as the tight fascia and muscles give up their long-held tension, a miraculous thing happens: our thoughts and spirit give up theirs as well.

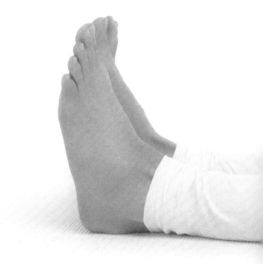

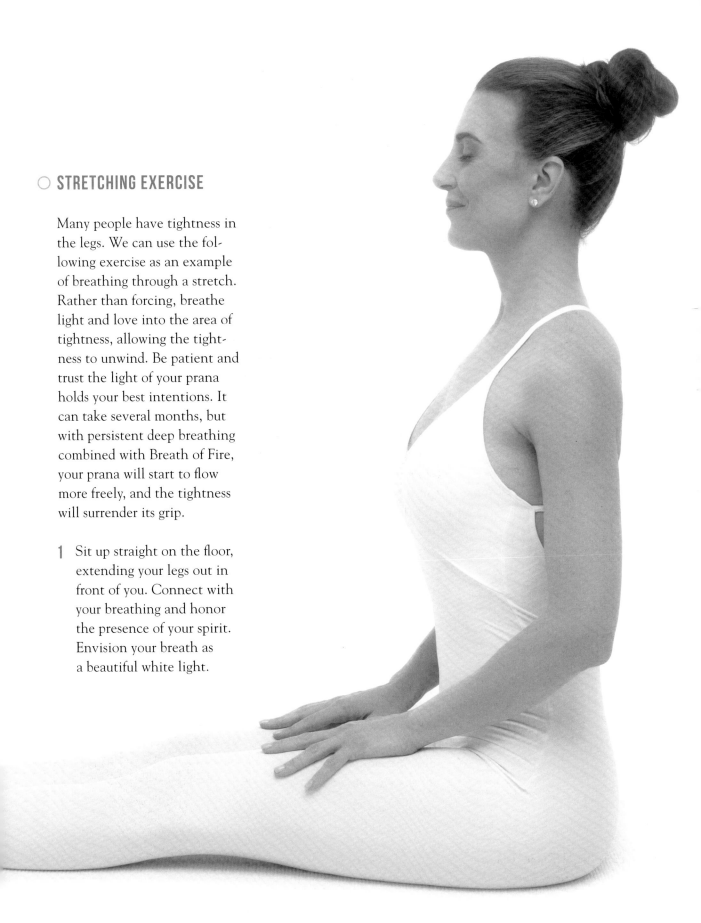

○ STRETCHING EXERCISE

Many people have tightness in the legs. We can use the following exercise as an example of breathing through a stretch. Rather than forcing, breathe light and love into the area of tightness, allowing the tightness to unwind. Be patient and trust the light of your prana holds your best intentions. It can take several months, but with persistent deep breathing combined with Breath of Fire, your prana will start to flow more freely, and the tightness will surrender its grip.

1 Sit up straight on the floor, extending your legs out in front of you. Connect with your breathing and honor the presence of your spirit. Envision your breath as a beautiful white light.

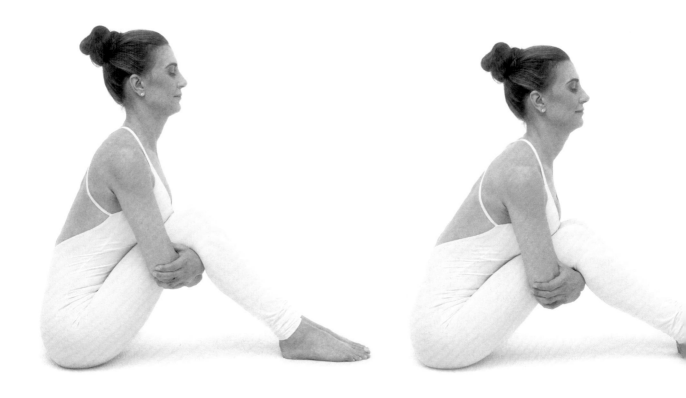

2 While inhaling and exhaling deeply, bend your knees, lift your thighs, and wrap your arms around the backs of your thighs, hugging them to you. Hinge forward from your hips so that your torso is pressed as closely as possible into your upper thighs. Keep your navel pointed forward and your neck relaxed. Continue inhaling deeply into your abdomen and fully exhaling all the air from your lungs.

3 As you breathe, gradually move your heels away from you so you hinge farther forward. Only move your heels forward to the extent that you can maintain the hug, with your thighs remaining pressed to your chest. Once you reach the point where your thighs and torso start to separate, stop and soften into the position and breathe deeply.

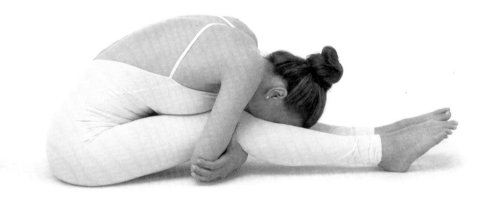

4 Continue taking long, slow breaths deeply into your abdomen. Try to breathe as profoundly as possible, remembering the four-part Square Breath as described in chapter 3. Envision your breath as light flowing through the areas of tightness in your lower spine or behind your legs. Continue for one to three minutes.

5 Practice Breath of Fire for an additional one to three minutes while continuing to visualize the flow of prana.

6 As your body begins to relax, you will find you can move your heels farther forward. Go ahead and move them, but keep your torso against your thighs. Be patient, relax, and focus on your breathing. Don't overdo it or strain. Be patient.

7 To finish, inhale very deeply, hold the position, then exhale fully, deepening into the stretch. Repeat the full inhalation and exhalation two more times; then relax onto your back. Allow the current of prana to be a river of love flowing through you.

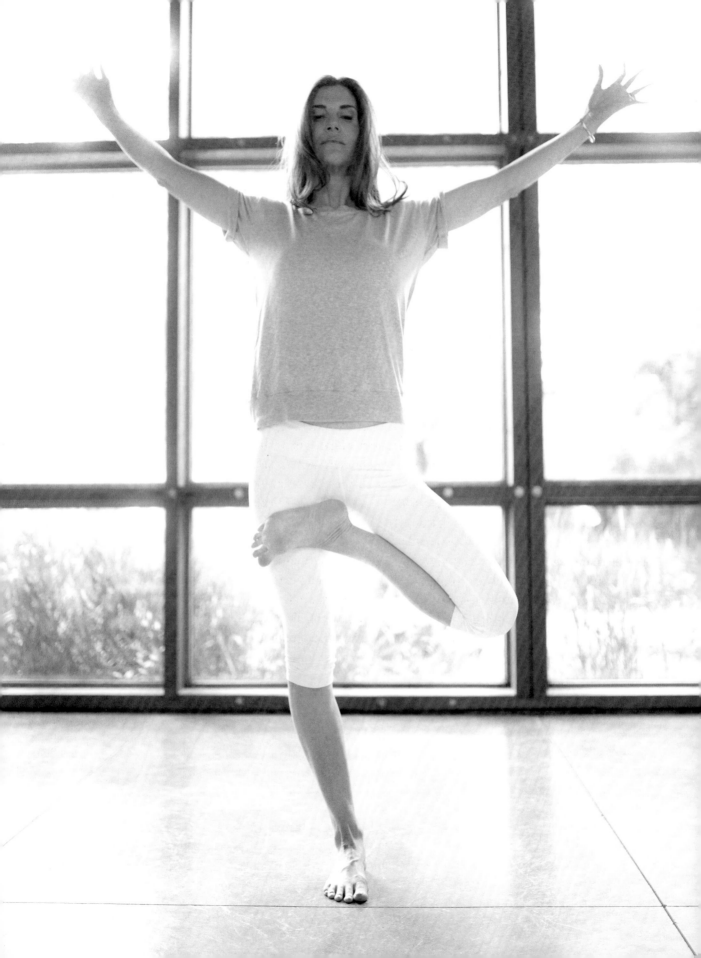

8 CLASSIC KUNDALINI YOGA SETS

THE CORE TECHNIQUES OF KUNDALINI yoga are the sequences of exercises called *sets*. These sequences are designed to stimulate our health response and optimize the flow and frequency of our energy. The sets and exercises in kundalini yoga are known as *kriyas* (pronounced "*kree*-yah"). Kriyas are groups of exercises that are practiced to produce a specific result. The kriyas of kundalini yoga were developed and refined over thousands of years in India. There are thousands of kriyas for everything from digestion to weight loss to prosperity.

For this chapter, we chose seven of our favorite sets for their ability to dissolve barriers and release the flow of prana through your body and your aura. They are extremely transformational. They are also simple enough for first-timers to dive into, but we still challenge ourselves with them after decades of practice.

GETTING THE MOST OUT OF THE SETS

These sets are especially effective because each exercise builds on the previous to generate a powerful shift in your energy field. To gain the effect, the sets and kriyas should be practiced in the order of exercises specified, from beginning to end. We invite you to choose one of these to immerse yourself in and to practice regularly for a period of forty days; then watch the transformation that opens up in your life.

We have made it a point to add the practice of tuning in with the Adi Mantra, use of an energy lock to complete most exercises, and Deep Relaxation at the end of every set, whether or not those elements were included in the original classes. Starting a kundalini yoga session by first tuning in with deep breathing and the Adi Mantra, then using the energy locks in your practice, and finishing with Deep Relaxation will integrate your health at cellular, energetic, and spiritual levels. These are the moments when true healing happens.

SPINAL ENERGY ACTIVATION

This classic kriya is one of the most powerful in kundalini yoga. It opens the energy centers along the spine so our prana can awaken and flow without restriction. It develops flexibility and brings oxygen to the discs between the vertebrae as well as opening up the fascia that can become chronically constricted in the back and between the ribs. It gives an internal massage to the cerebrospinal fluid, bringing nutrients into and removing toxins from stagnant areas of the brain. Moving the cerebrospinal fluid up the spine with the action of the exercises in this set helps bring balance to our neurotransmitters. When our neurotransmitters are not in balance, we can become depressed or anxious, or we find we either are tired all the time or cannot sleep at night. When our neurotransmitters are balanced, however, we experience bliss. The locks in this sequence cause kundalini energy to flow through the spine, awakening the chakras.

With ongoing, steady practice of this set, your spine becomes limber, fills with a beautiful light, and feels wonderfully luminous. That light in our spine is who we are, much more so than the bones and cartilage of the physical spine.

1 TUNE IN

1 Sit with a straight spine in a cross-legged position. Close your eyes, inhale and exhale profoundly, and bring your attention to your breath flowing deeply into the core of your being.

2 Chant the Adi Mantra three or more times. For more on the Adi Mantra, please refer to chapter 6.

Ong

Namo

Guru

Dev

Namo

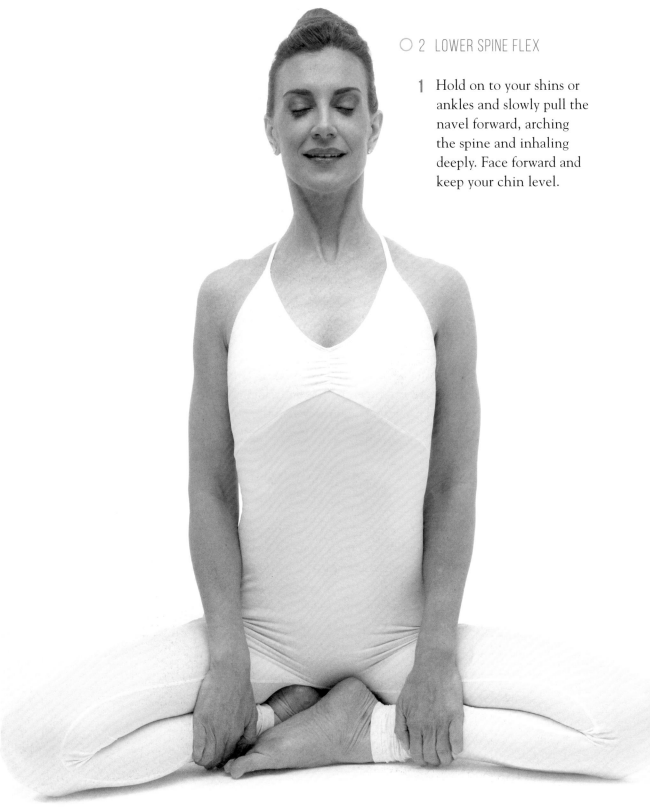

2 LOWER SPINE FLEX

1 Hold on to your shins or ankles and slowly pull the navel forward, arching the spine and inhaling deeply. Face forward and keep your chin level.

2 Exhale as you flex the spine backward, drawing the navel straight back and tucking the abdomen in.

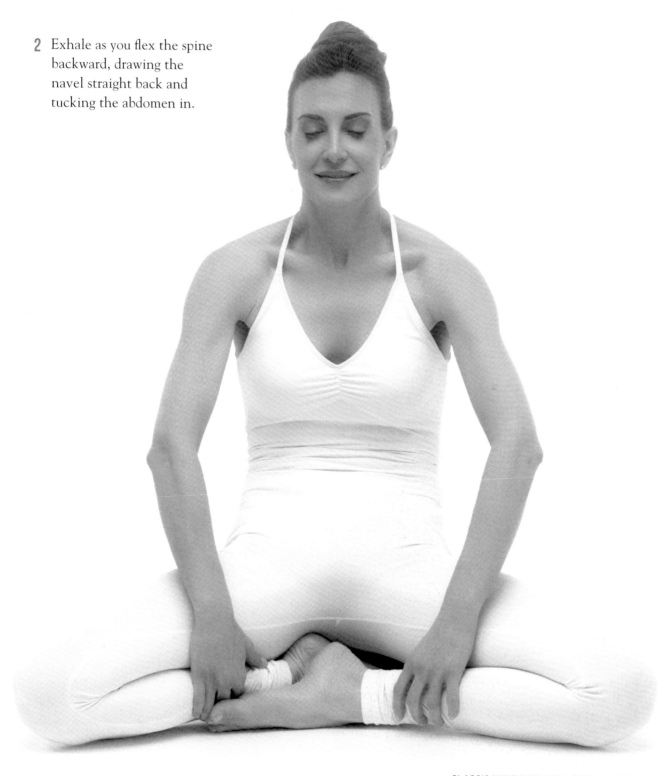

3 Continue moving your lower spine, inhaling as you flex forward and exhaling as you flex back. Start slowly, feeling the full extent of the pull and noticing where your body holds your resistance. Deepen into the movement, and as your spine warms up, go a little faster. If you are feeling into it, you can flex quite fast and intensely. No matter what your speed is, flex completely forward and all the way back, consciously and with awareness. Inhale as you expand your rib cage and move your heart forward and exhale as you move your heart back. Continue flexing for 26 to 108 repetitions.

4 To finish, sit up tall and inhale deeply. Draw breath deeply into your abdomen, filling your lungs and expanding your rib cage. Suspend the breath while applying Root Lock and Neck Lock. Hold for as long as you feel comfortable and, when ready, slowly let the air out, but keep the internal focus. Hold the breath out as you apply Maha Bhand. Then inhale and exhale naturally. Sit for one minute and feel the change in your energy.

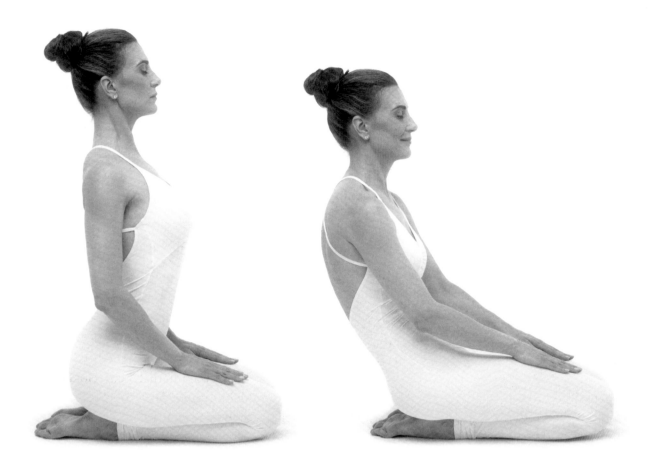

○ 3 MIDSPINE FLEX

The second exercise is similar to the first, but sitting in a new position, with the heels beneath the buttocks, stimulates the life nerve and allows for maximum flexion slightly higher up the spinal column. The core of the body, internal organs, and navel point become energized.

1 Sit on the floor in a kneeling position, with the heels beneath the buttocks and your hands on your thighs, palms down.

2 Close your eyes and inhale as you flex your spine, drawing your navel straight forward.

3 Flex backward as you exhale. Keep your chin level and facing forward rather than tipping the head.

4 Continue moving your navel forward and backward with your breath. Begin slowly, really tuning in to the stretch, and then increase your speed as you feel comfortable. Repeat 26 to 108 times.

5 To finish, sit up tall, inhale deeply, suspend the breath, and apply Root Lock and Neck Lock. We invite you to visualize your energy as a white light rising up the center of your spine. When you feel ready, exhale slowly then sit and breathe gently for two minutes, and feel your body glowing.

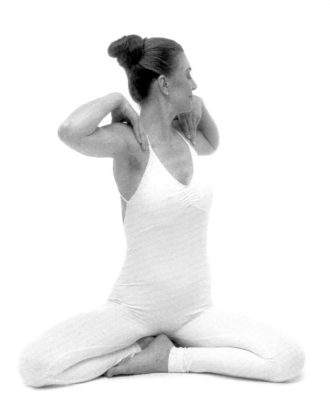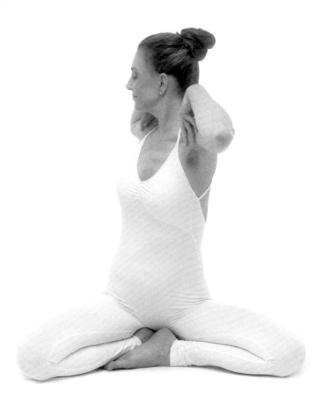

○ 4 WASHING MACHINE

This exercise lifts prana from the third to the fourth chakra.

1 Sit in a cross-legged position. Close your eyes and feel your spine rising up like the stalk of a tall flower, sensing the energy pathway from the pelvis to the top of the head.

2 Holding this awareness, lift both elbows out to each side and place your hands on your shoulders, right hand on right shoulder and left on left, with the fingers in front and thumbs behind.

3 With a steady, fluid movement, on the inhale twist your torso all the way to the left, and on the exhale twist to the right. Keep twisting, led by your breath and swinging the elbows from side to side, letting the momentum carry you smoothly. Repeat twenty-six times.

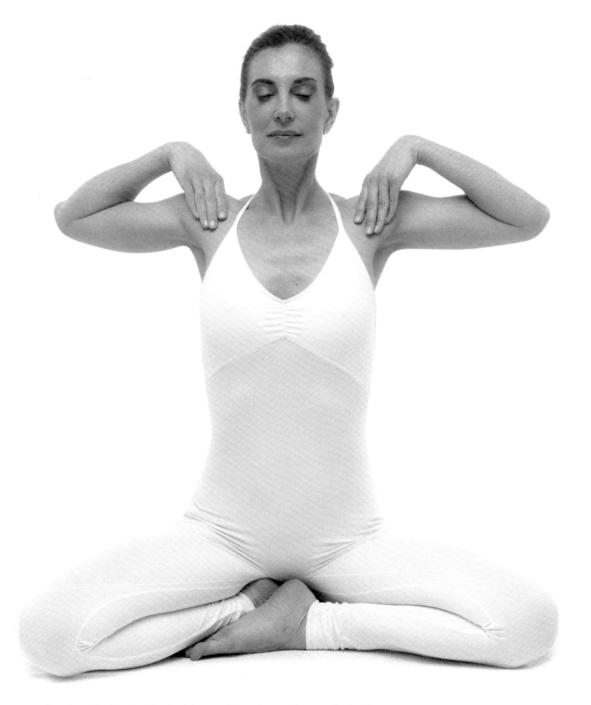

4 To finish, inhale deeply, hold your breath in, then exhale the breath out as you relax. Inhale again and apply Root Lock and Neck Lock. Hold for as long as you can while perceiving your energy rising through your rib cage. When you release the breath, hold on to the awareness you have gained.

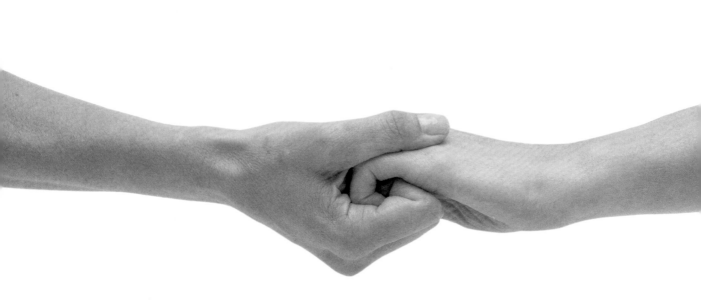

○ 5 BEAR GRIP AT HEART CENTER

The fourth exercise of this set clears and energizes our heart chakra. This sacred pathway of shifting our energy from the navel to the heart is one of the most profound journeys of life.

1 Sit in a cross-legged position with your hands in Bear Grip. Hold your left hand in front of your chest with the thumb down and palm facing forward. Hold your right palm in front of the left with palm facing back and thumb up. Curl the fingers of both hands, hook them together tightly, and pull your elbows firmly to the sides. The fingers should remain hooked together. Pull hard but don't let go.

2 Swivel your elbows up and down with an alternating seesaw movement, keeping your hands in Bear Grip. As you lift the right elbow, the left elbow goes down, and as you lift the left, the right goes down. Exhale rapidly each time an elbow comes up, practicing Breath of Fire in rhythm with the fast movement. Continue for one to three minutes.

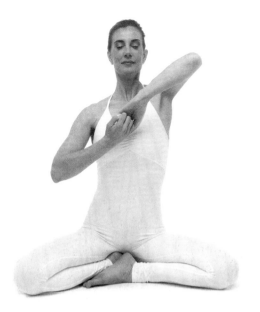

3 Inhale deeply into your abdomen, then exhale completely, fully emptying the lungs. With your breath held out, pull on the hands as hard as you can, drawing in on the navel point. Apply Maha Bhand.

4 When you feel you are ready to inhale, take a deep, conscious breath. Then exhale again and repeat the pull on Bear Grip. Repeat Maha Bhand while pulling forcefully on Bear Grip up to three times total.

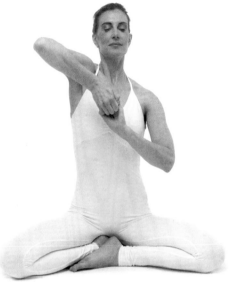

5 Let the hands come to rest on the knees. Breathe gently yet deeply, tuning in to the flow of energy into your heart center for thirty seconds.

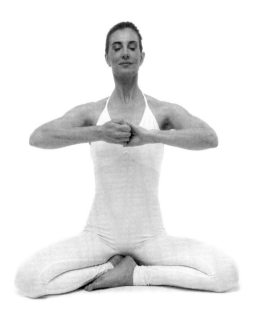

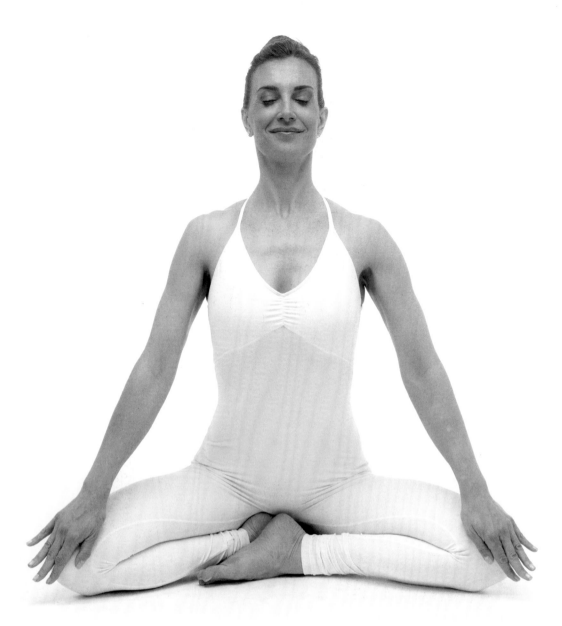

○ 6 UPPER SPINE FLEX

1 Sit in a cross-legged
position and hold on to
your knees with your elbows
as straight as possible.

2 As you inhale, flex your
chest and upper spine
forward, pulling back on
the knees and feeling
your rib cage expand.

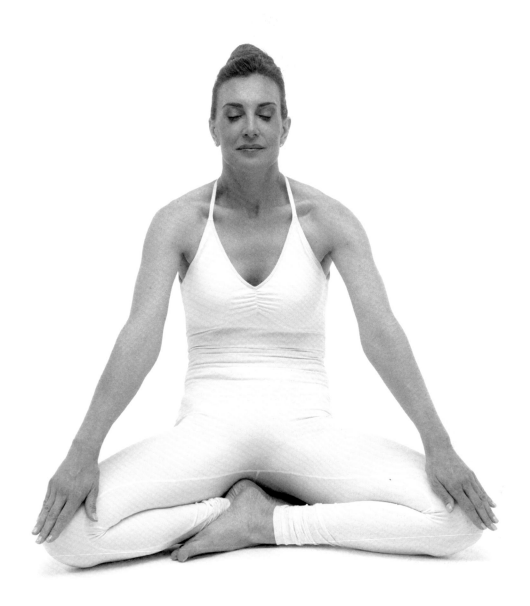

3 As you exhale, flex your upper spine backward into an arch. Try to focus the movement on the upper spine and rib cage. Keep your chin and neck steady rather than bobbing up and down.

4 Repeat the back-and-forth spine flexion 26 to 108 times, letting your breath lead the movement.

5 To finish, sit up straight, inhale into the depths of your belly, suspend your breath, and apply Root Lock and Neck Lock.

6 Let your breath return to a normal rhythm. Relax in a seated position for one minute, sensing the inner flow of your own energy.

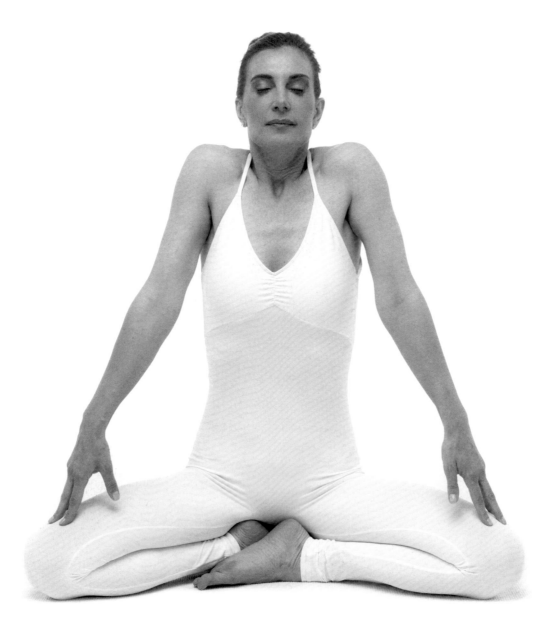

○ 7 SHOULDER SHRUGS

1 Sit in a cross-legged
position with your hands
on your knees and shoulders
loose and relaxed.

2 Inhale and raise
both shoulders up to
toward your ears.

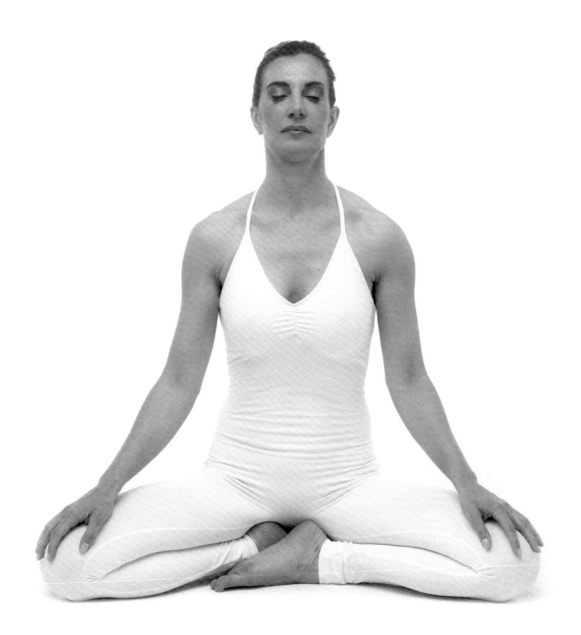

3 As you exhale, let the shoulders release and drop down fully, as though they were dangling.

4 Continue lifting and releasing the shoulders about once per second,

for less than two minutes total. Feel your tension and restriction sloughing off.

5 To finish, inhale and lift both shoulders. Hold the breath in and the shoulders lifted for fifteen

seconds. Slowly release with an exhale. Continue sitting, breathing, and tuning in to the beauty of the energy that flows through and around you.

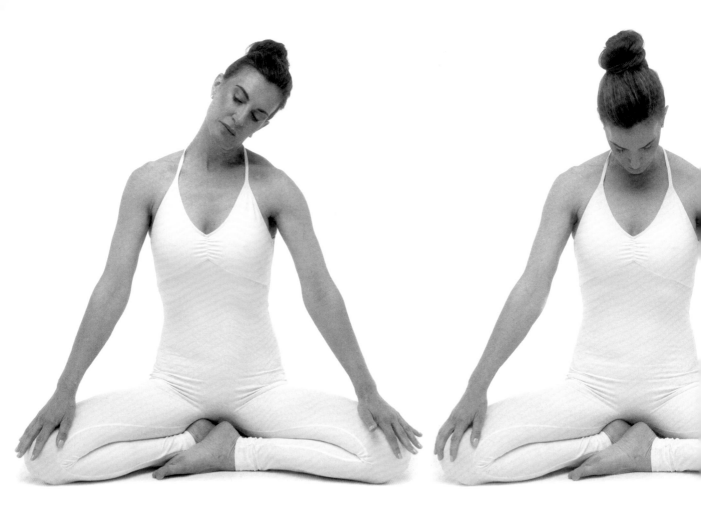

○ 8 NECK ROLLS

1 Sit up straight. Allow the chin to slowly drop forward onto
  the chest, feeling the stretch in the back of the neck.

2 Slowly roll your left ear toward your right shoulder, feeling
  the stretch on the right side of the neck. Drop the head
  back and then roll your right ear toward your left shoulder.

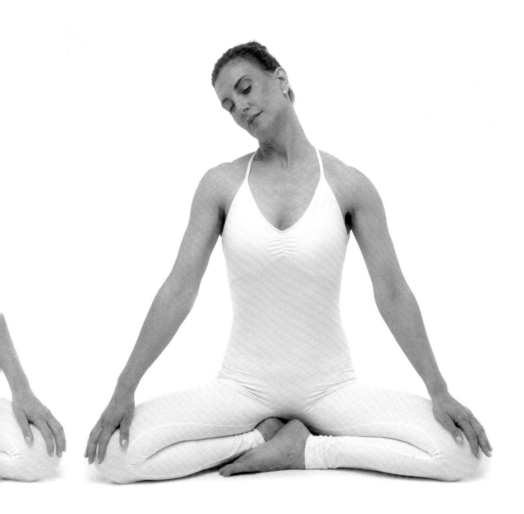

3 Continue rotating the neck by moving the chin in large circles for five repetitions. Go slowly, deeply feeling the stretch. Then reverse direction and repeat the action the same number of times on the other side.

4 To finish, bring your head up straight, breathe full, deep breaths, and focus on your third eye point.

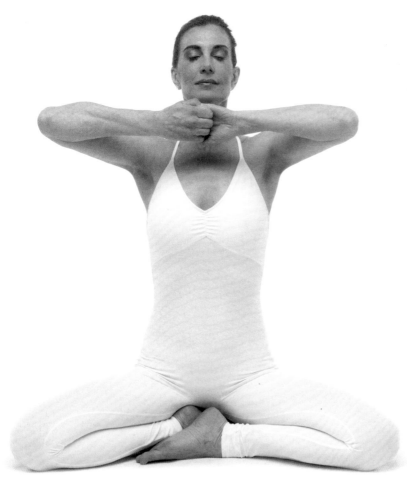

○ 9 BEAR GRIP PITUITARY ACTIVATION

1 Sit up straight and tall. With your elbows out, bring your fingers into Bear Grip again, but this time in front of your throat.

2 Inhale deeply and hold the breath. Maintain Bear Grip and pull your elbows to the sides as hard as you can. Pull powerfully for five to fifteen seconds while holding the breath in and concentrating on your third eye point.

3 Fully exhale while holding the same position and concentrating on the third eye point. With the breath held out again, pull as hard as you can on Bear Grip for five to fifteen seconds.

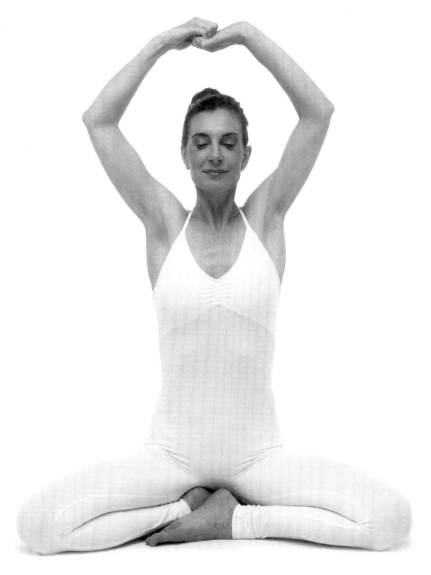

4 Inhale as you lift Bear Grip
   six inches over the top of
   your head. Hold your breath
   in and pull strongly on
   Bear Grip, concentrating
   your attention at the
   very top of your head, for
   five to fifteen seconds.

5 Stay in the position and
   exhale completely, fully
   emptying the lungs.

Holding your breath out,
again pull on the grip
overhead, focusing on
the top of the head, for
five to fifteen seconds.

6 As you inhale, return
   your Bear Grip to the area
   in front of your throat.
   Repeat the sequence two
   more times, inhaling and
   exhaling with Bear Grip

in front of the throat, then
inhaling and exhaling with
Bear Grip overhead, as
described in steps 2 to 6.

7 To finish, allow your hands
   to come down to rest on
   your knees. Breathe with
   awareness and feel the shifts
   in your subtle flow of energy.

1   Sit on your heels with your spine tall. Draw your chin back slightly so your neck is in Neck Lock. Reach your arms straight up overhead with the elbows alongside your ears. Interlock all your fingers together, keeping only the index fingers stretched straight up and pressed together.

Sat Nam

2   Draw the navel sharply in toward your spine as you say the mantra "Sat" out loud. Then, release the navel and say the mantra, "Nam" out loud.

3   Continue to draw the navel sharply in on each "Sat," and release it on each "Nam" with a steady rhythm slightly slower than one per second. Allow your breath to come and go as feels natural. Continue for three to thirty-one minutes.

4   To finish, inhale as deeply into your abdomen while holding the arm position. Hold the breath, pull back on the navel, focus at your third eye point, and squeeze the energy through the central channel of the spine to the top of your head. We invite you to feel a bright, white light flowing through your spine and out the top of the head toward your fingertips. Exhale, then repeat a second time.

5   Inhale, exhale, and hold the breath out. Apply the Maha Bhand, focusing at your third eye point, and again draw energy up your spine and out the top of head.

6   To end, inhale, exhale, bring your arms down to rest on your thighs, and breathe normally. We invite you to feel your spine as luminous and divine. For additional details and a photo of Sat Kriya, please see page 125-127.

11 DEEP RELAXATION

Relax on your back for fifteen minutes, and allow your body and spirit to assimilate the practice you've just done. Feel the glow around you as it heals the energy you are clearing. If there are any walls remaining around you, allow them to dissolve at this time. Deep Relaxation is the most important part of this kriya. Continue to focus on the golden glow around you—you are like a shining sun projecting rays of light in all directions. Be still and know you are manifesting your dreams as you rest.

THE PITUITARY GLAND SERIES FOR INTUITION

The pituitary gland is the master gland, controlling the hormones of the entire body, working in conjunction with our nerves to build balance, and opening the gates of our awareness. When our pituitary is awakened, our consciousness awakens as well. Our nerves open to increased levels of high-frequency energy, we become aware of the presence of the divine within us, and our intuition blossoms. This is a powerful set and one of our all-time favorites.

1 TUNE IN

1 Sit up tall and feel the flow of breath through your nostrils. Sense an energetic connection between your navel and mother earth below.

2 Place your palms together in Prayer Pose and feel the flow of energy moving in and out of you with your breath. When you feel ready, chant the Adi Mantra three or more times.

Ong
Namo
Guru
Dev
Namo

○ 2 HIGH LUNGE

1 From the standing position, come into a lunge by bending your right knee and extending your left leg straight out behind you; stabilize the leg on the ball of the left foot. Bend your torso forward and place your fingertips on the floor alongside your body for balance. Elongate your neck, look straight ahead, and expand your rib cage by lifting the ribs away from the intercostal muscles. Place your right knee directly over your right ankle. Lift your chin to activate the line of energy extending from your left heel to the point between your eyebrows.

2 Hold this lunge and breathe deeply into the lowermost part of your body, as though you could draw breath all the way to the tips of your toes. Continue holding and breathing deeply for fifteen seconds to one full minute.

3 Stay in the lunge position and begin Breath of Fire as described in chapter 4. Continue for fifteen seconds to two minutes.

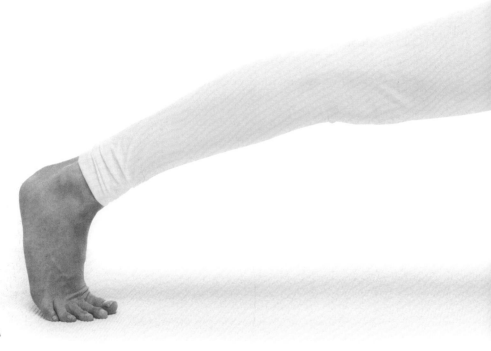

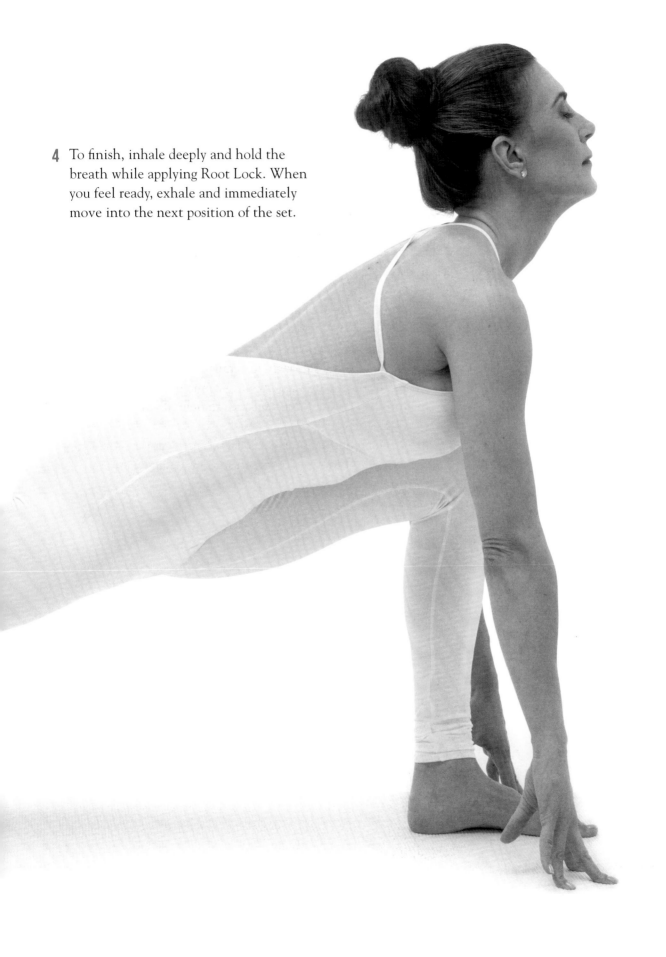

4 To finish, inhale deeply and hold the breath while applying Root Lock. When you feel ready, exhale and immediately move into the next position of the set.

1 Using your hands to support your weight, carefully lower your right shin and knee onto the floor, allowing your right foot to scoot back toward the left hip until you find the right position for your level of flexibility. Bring your navel forward and fold your torso down over your right leg, resting your belly against the right thigh. Continue bringing your forehead down until it rests on the ground or on a folded blanket in front of the right leg.

Once you are in the basic Lunge Rest and feel comfortable enough, settle into it more deeply by taking the weight off your hands and folding them back alongside your body with the palms facing up. Relax your shoulders. Keep the left leg fully extended behind you with the top of the foot on the ground. Surrender your muscles to gravity.

After you are settled in, the key is to breathe as slowly and fully as possibly, drawing prana into your abdomen and back to your left toes. Feel light and loving energy flowing through the areas of resistance, washing away the tension, running through your thighs, and releasing the blockages.

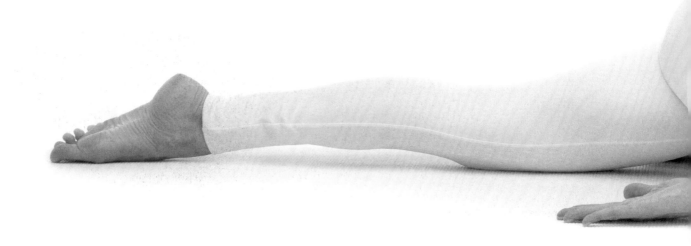

Visualize a powerful purple light just between your eyebrows while pressing your forehead into the floor or a folded blanket. Stay in the position for twenty seconds to three minutes.

2 Remain in this position for one to four minutes. Practice long, deep breathing as you surrender and bring a new balance to the hormones that are secreting throughout your physical body.

3 To finish, exhale fully and, with the breath held out, apply Root Lock. When you feel ready, inhale and come out of the position.

4 Repeat the previous two positions, High Lunge and Lunge Rest, on the other side of your body, starting with the lunge onto the left foot.

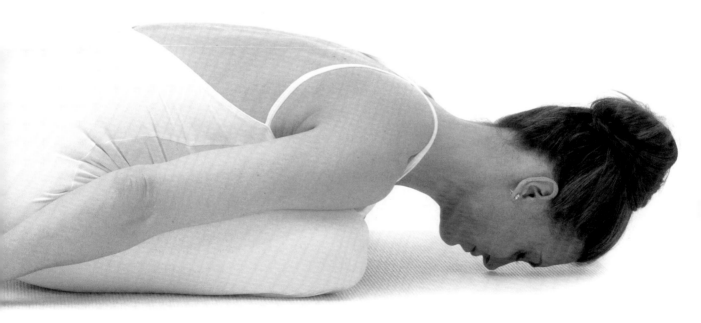

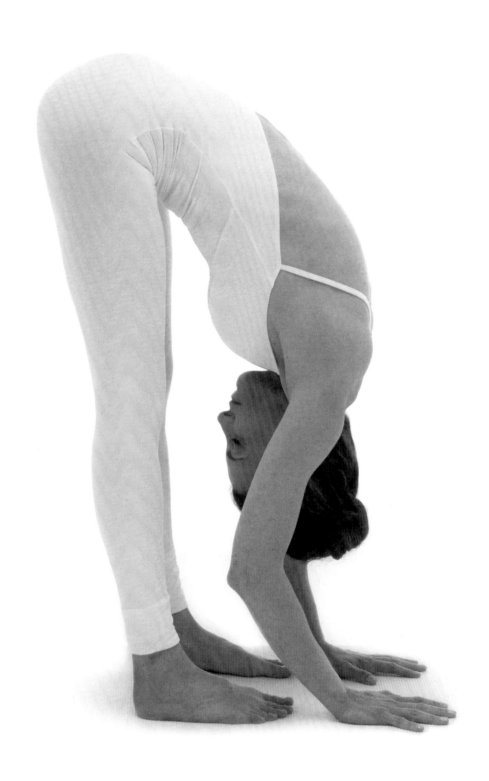

○ 4 STANDING FORWARD BEND

1 Stand up straight with your feet shoulder width apart. Feel your spine rising tall from your pelvis to the top of your head. Relax your shoulders and let your arms dangle at your sides.

2 Bending from your hips, hinge your torso forward and bring your navel down toward your thighs, keeping your buttocks pushed back. Continue bending forward and down, releasing your spine so that it simply dangles and surrenders to gravity. Allow your arms and neck to dangle freely as well.

3 Continue relaxing into the position for one to four minutes. Breathe deeply into your abdomen, feeling the expansion and contraction of the rib cage with every breath. We invite you to direct the light of your breath to wash through the areas of tightness and energetic blocks. This position helps balance your nervous system and permits you to surrender your thoughts.

4 To come out of the position, bend your knees slightly, tuck your tailbone, and begin straightening your spine. Starting from the lowermost vertebrae, lift first your lower spine, then your midspine, and finally your upper spine. Your neck and head should come up last. Feel yourself standing tall, with your spinal column aligned and radiant.

○ 5 STANDING V ARMS

1 Stand up tall with your feet shoulder width apart. Curl
your fingers into the mounds at the base of your fingers and
straighten your thumbs away from the rest of your fingers.

2 Lift and spread your arms, creating a V shape overhead, with
the thumbs pointing straight up and your other fingers still
curled in. Breathe slowly and deeply, fully filling your lungs
on the inhale and emptying them completely on the exhale.
Keep your spine elongated and feel the pressure of your breath
against your spine. Envision a line of energy running from your
heart through your shoulders and from your elbows to your
thumbs. Continue for forty-five seconds to three minutes.

3 To finish, inhale deeply and hold your breath as
long as you feel comfortable while applying Root
Lock. Exhale and relax out of the position.

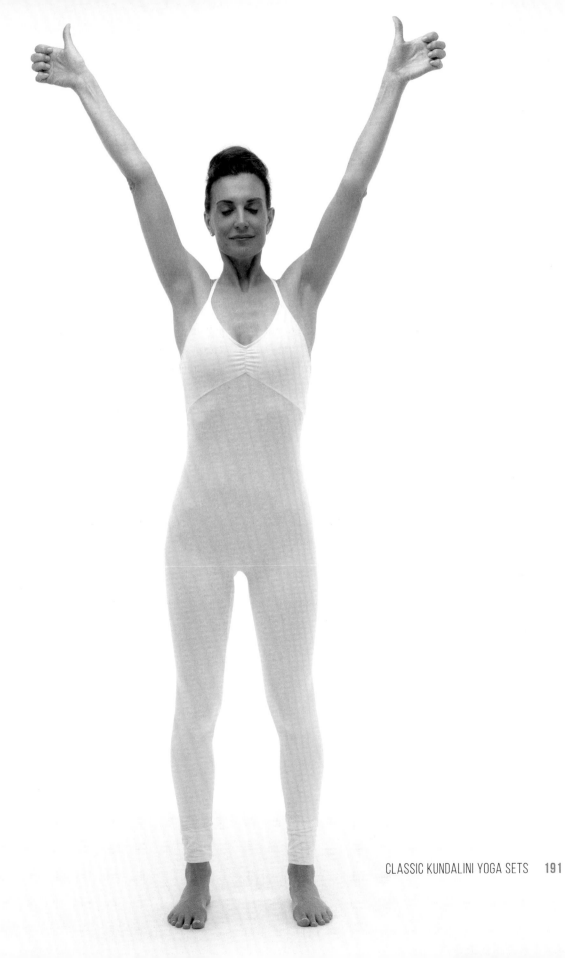

1 Stand up tall with your feet shoulder width apart. Bend your knees and, with fingers spread wide, place your palms on the floor one leg's length in front you. Support your weight evenly between your hands and feet.

2 Straighten your legs, bringing your buttocks up high and hinging from the hip joints rather than the waist. Melt your heart toward the earth and soften your belly while you deepen your breathing. Hold the pose and breathe deeply for forty-five seconds to three minutes.

3 To finish, inhale deeply and hold the breath in. Then exhale and bring your knees down to come out of the position, preparing yourself to lie on your belly.

MODIFICATION 1 Place a rolled-up towel or yoga mat or a folded blanket beneath your heels.

MODIFICATION 2 Come down onto all fours with your knees on the ground for the entire pose.

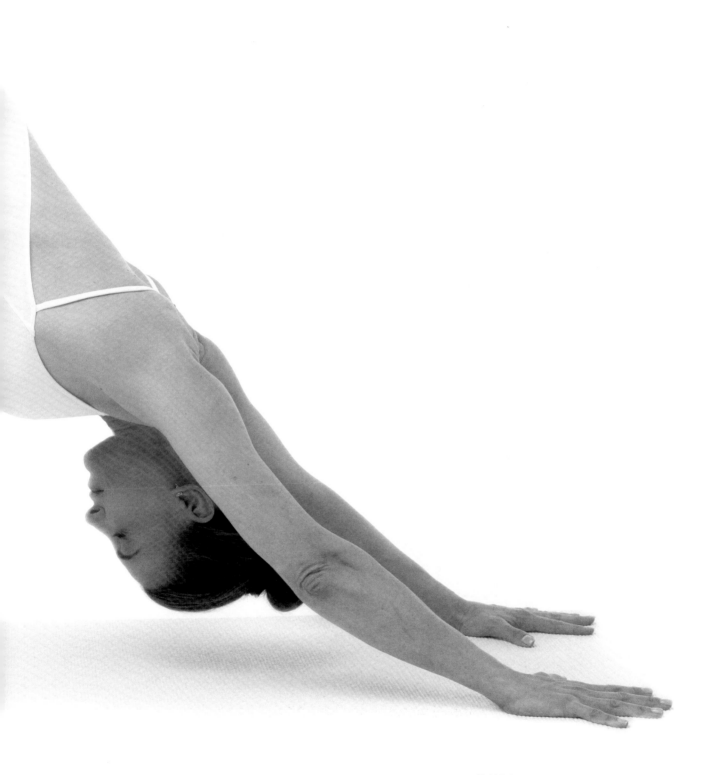

○ 7 COBRA NECK TWISTS

1 Lie down on your stomach. Relax with your forehead
   on the ground and your arms next to your body.
   Rest this way for one minute while integrating the
   posture and rebalancing your glandular system.

2 Still lying on your stomach, press your palms into the
   ground just below your shoulders and lift your heart up.
   Lift your chin up and stretch your head back to feel a deep
   expansion through your chest. Breathe deeply for one
   minute in this Cobra Pose, softening at the heart center.
   Keep your shoulders down and heels close together.

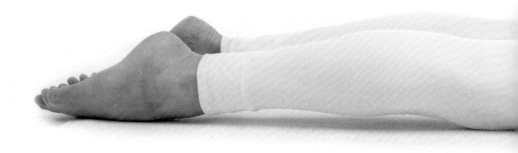

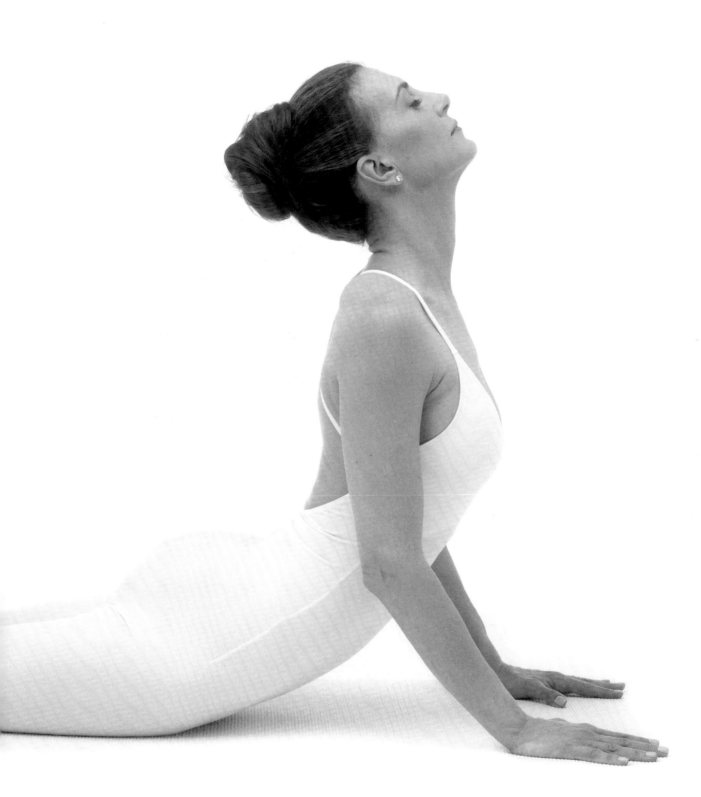

3 Maintaining the position, inhale as you turn your head to the left shoulder and exhale as you turn your head to the right shoulder. Continue this head movement and breath pattern for thirty seconds to two minutes.

4 Still holding Cobra Pose, inhale and suspend the breath while applying Root Lock. Exhale and release the lock. Repeat two more times.

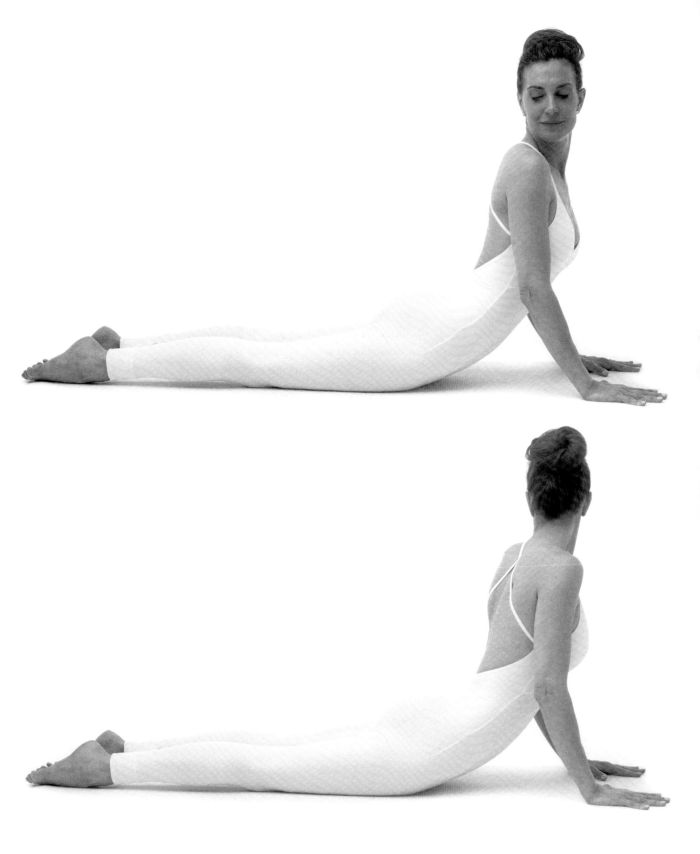

○ 8 FLOWER BLOSSOM

1   Sit on your heels and spread your knees apart. Bring
your palms to the floor at the sides of your hips.
Draw your forehead down toward the floor as you exhale.

2   Inhale as you lift your buttocks up off your heels. While lifting
your torso, reach your arms straight up to the sky and open
them wide until your thighs are straight and perpendicular to
the floor. Your shins remain on the ground. Imagine yourself
as a beautiful flower bathing in the warmth of the sun as
your petals open. Be careful to not overextend your back.

3   Exhale and close your petals as you relax down and
come back into the original seated position with your
knees open. Inhale and open up; exhale and close down.
Continue for forty-five seconds to three minutes.

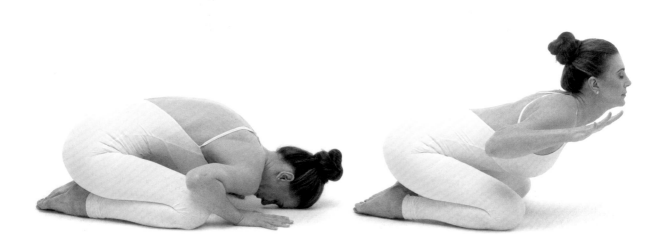

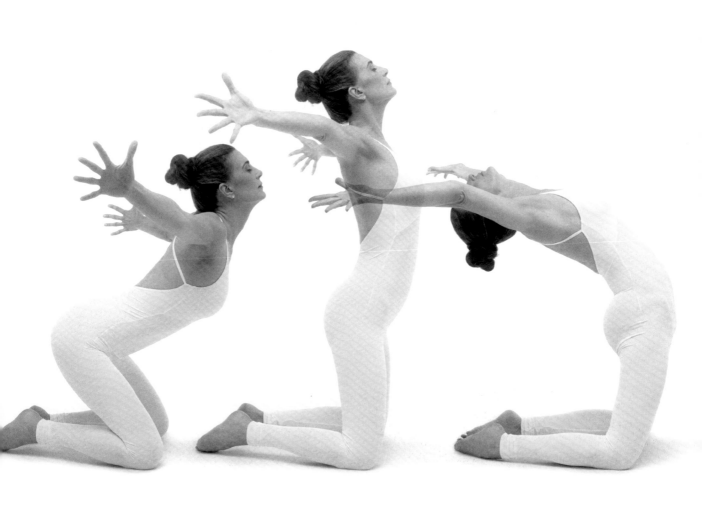

○ 9 YOGA MUDRA

1 Remain seated on your heels, with your spine tall. Interlace your fingers in Venus Lock behind you. Hinging from your hips, draw your navel forward toward your thighs.

2 Continue hinging forward and down, elongating your spine, with the neck and head at last coming to rest on the ground in front of you. Draw your arms up toward the sky behind you, keeping your fingers interlaced. Bring your arms back as far as possible as you draw your forehead back toward the earth. Take long, slow breaths while holding the position for one to three minutes.

○ 10 DEEP RELAXATION

Come to rest on your back. Completely surrender in Deep Relaxation after this set while the wisdom of your body takes over. Lie down onto your back with palms face up alongside your body. Allow your soul to connect with your breathing, thoughts, and physical body as your hormones regulate naturally. You have just completed a magical set. Enjoy your peace.

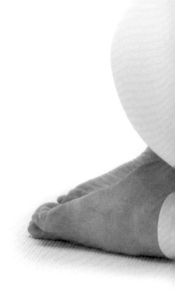

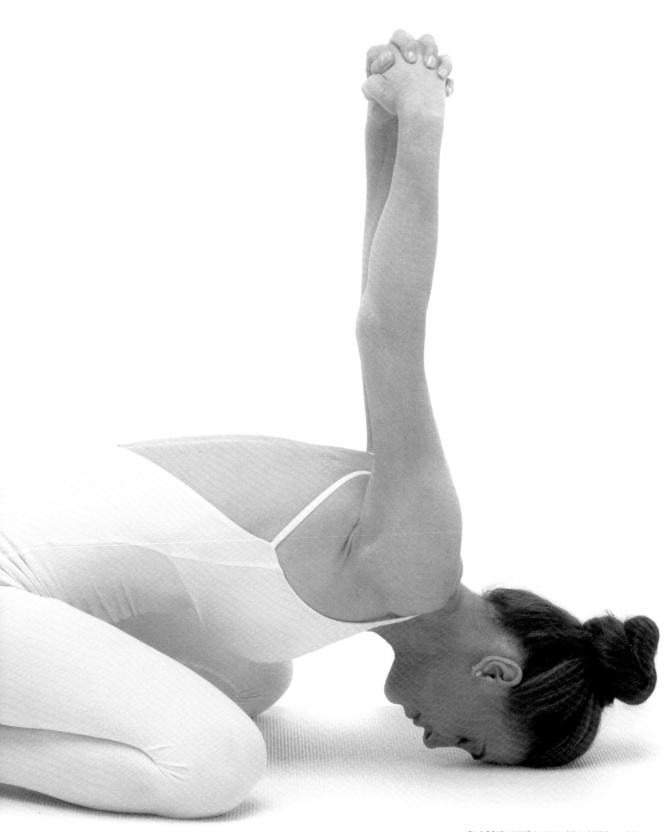

YOGA FOR THE SPINE AND IMMUNE SYSTEM

This yoga set removes the fog from and opens the body's central channel of energy, the sushmana. The sushmana is the main avenue of light that follows the pathway of the spine, and this set acts like the morning street sweeper clearing away debris so our energy can flow with delight. When that light is bright, moving without blocks, and shining with the frequency of love, we can sparkle our radiance out to the ends of the universe. This set also promotes a lot of flexibility, integrating spirit and spine together to activate your fullest potential.

○ 1 TUNE IN

Ong
Namo
Guru
Dev
Namo

1 Sit in a cross-legged position and slow your breathing down. Feel the breath flowing deeply into your abdomen and your rib cage, expanding them with each inhale.

2 While continuing to breathe deeply, press your palms together in front of your heart and chant the Adi Mantra three or more times.

○ 2 SPINAL TWIST

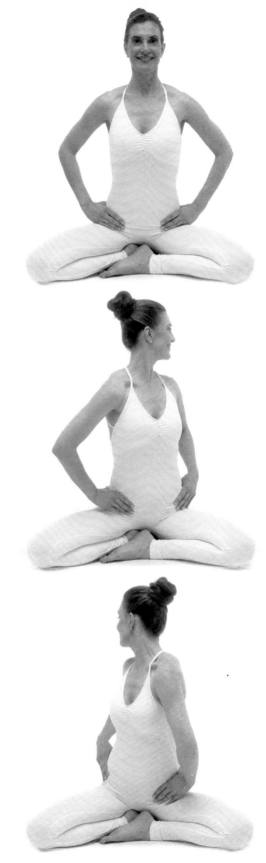

1 Sit up with a straight spine. Place your hands on either side of your waist, with thumbs in back, fingers in front, and elbows out to the sides. Feel the flow of breath coming deeply into your abdomen.

2 Begin twisting your torso to the left and right in a fluid and meditative motion, exhaling to each side and inhaling as you pass the center. Keep your spine tall. As your spine warms up, you can increase the pace until you are being carried by the momentum. Continue for one to five minutes.

3 To finish, return to the center position and inhale deeply. Exhale and, while holding your breath out, apply Maha Bhand again. Then inhale and transition to normal breathing.

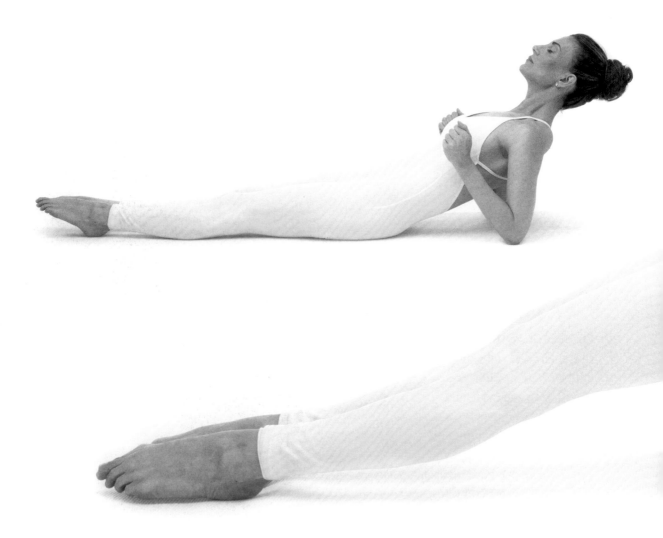

○ 3 BACK PLATFORM ON ELBOWS

1   Sit on the floor with your legs extended straight out in
front of you. Then lean back, supporting your weight with
your elbows pressed to the floor behind you. You may
wish to put a blanket beneath your elbows for padding.

2   Begin lifting and lowering your pelvis as you breathe
with Breath of Fire. To go up, press your heels and
elbows down hard to arch your back and lift the
buttocks off your mat. The Breath of Fire is continuous
and can be done at a faster pace than the lifts.

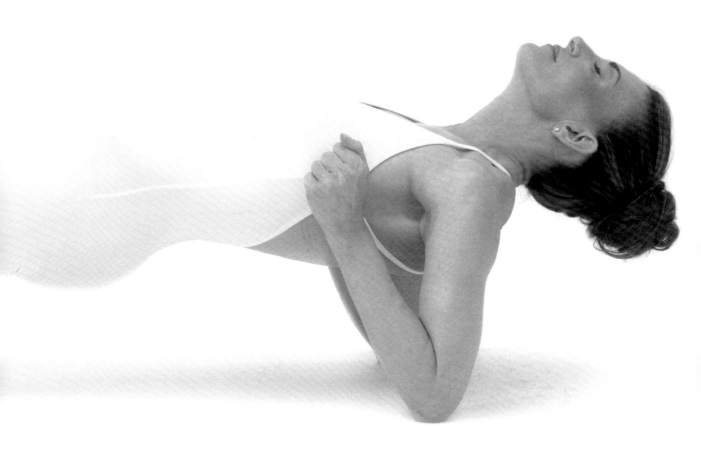

MODIFICATION To make the hip lifts less strenuous, bend your knees and bring your heels closer to your buttocks. The closer your heels are to your hips, the easier it is to lift them. If you still cannot lift your hips, press the elbows down as firmly as you can and practice Breath of Fire.

3 Continue raising and lowering your body while doing Breath of Fire for thirty seconds to three minutes.

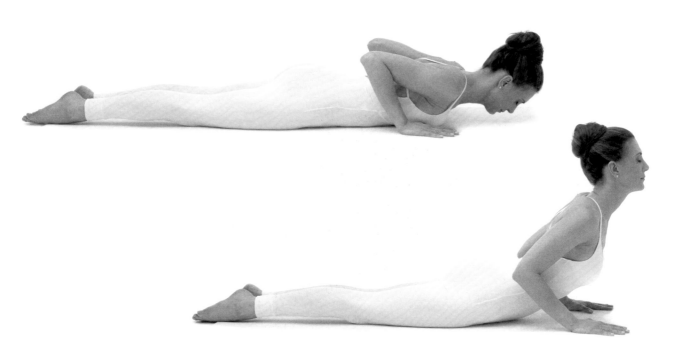

○ 4 COBRA FLEXES

1 Lie down flat on your stomach with your chin on the ground. Place your palms face down just below your shoulders.

2 Lift your chin off the mat and curl your neck back. Supporting your weight with your arms, continue curling your spine back and up, vertebra by vertebra, until you are in a back bend with chin lifted high.

3 Supporting your weight on your hands and toes, begin raising and lowering your torso as you do Breath of Fire. Pace yourself so the movement is slower than the breath. Continue for one to fifteen minutes.

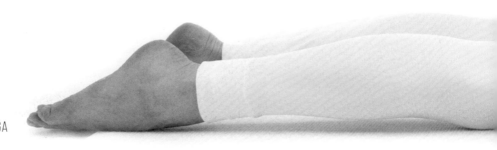

4 Inhale very deeply while you hold the up position. Hold the breath in and apply Root Lock.

5 Remaining in the up position, exhale fully. Apply Root Lock with your breath expelled.

6 Repeat steps 4 and 5 for a total of three cycles. Then very slowly inhale in the up position and exhale as you lower yourself, vertebra by vertebra, back down to the ground.

7 To finish, relax onto your stomach, turn a cheek to one side, and return to normal breathing. Allow your breath to flow freely.

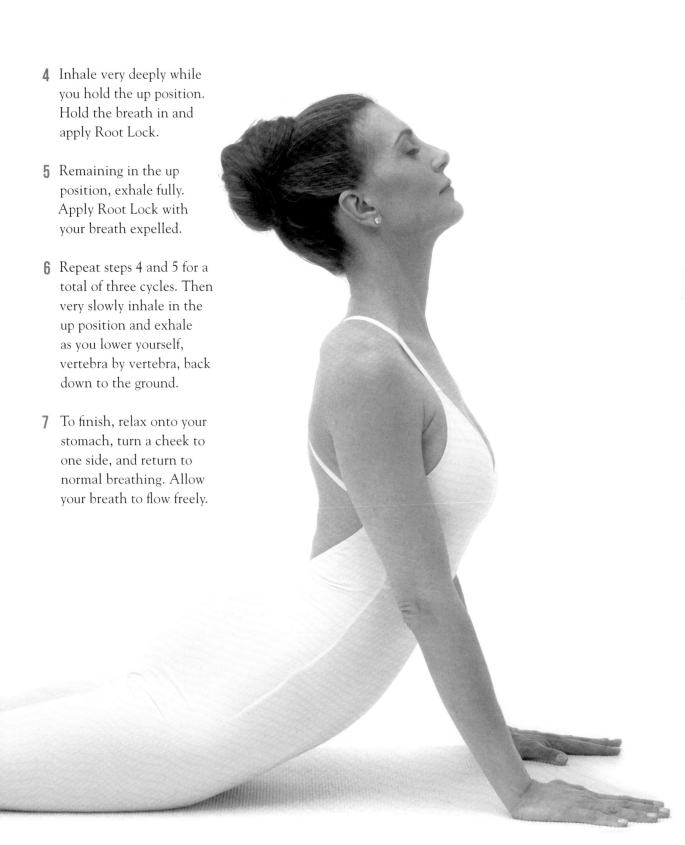

Rest on your back. Allow yourself to completely surrender in Deep Relaxation while you free yourself of blocks that were stuck in your spine. Honor yourself for doing this work and taking care of you. Your spine is the home of your immune system. Giving yourself this time to nourish and heal is extremely efficacious.

KRIYA FOR GOING WITH THE FLOW

Once we trust that everything happening to us in life is happening for a specific reason, we know we are in the flow. This does not mean that each moment of life is filled with bliss. It means that everything is in perfect, divine order, regardless of what it looks like on the outside. We recognize that the universe has its own intelligence and that all that happens in our personal lives is part of the larger divine dance.

We can control the circumstances of our life in exact proportion to the degree to which we can hold our breath—in other words, only a little while, compared to the vastness of all the breaths we take. God does all the rest, and just as we have to trust that the next breath will come, we can learn to trust that God is bringing us exactly what we need.

The following is a wonderful yoga set that shifts our energy and develops our ability to flow in all circumstances. It moves us into acceptance and allowing, peace and stillness. You may internally notice a shift at one point as you breathe through these poses. It just comes. This set uses parallel and perpendicular angles to balance and stream the earthly and heavenly energies through your nerves. The key is to keep your spine straight. In each of the four exercises, close your eyes, connect deeply with the breathing, and keep your body steady. Notice how your ribs are expanding and contracting as you breathe and how the inhale and exhale change the feel of the posture. Always stay connected to your heart beating in the center of it all.

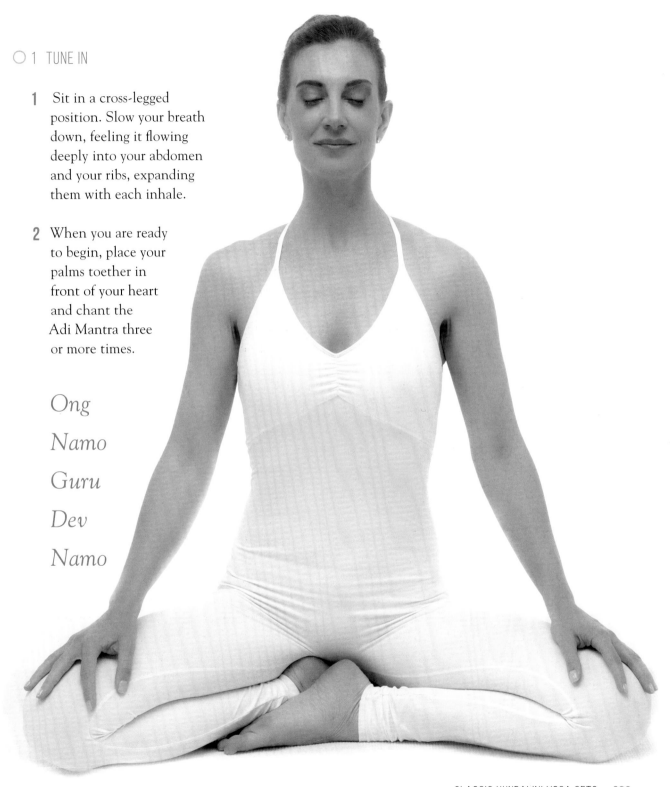

1 TUNE IN

1 Sit in a cross-legged position. Slow your breath down, feeling it flowing deeply into your abdomen and your ribs, expanding them with each inhale.

2 When you are ready to begin, place your palms toether in front of your heart and chant the Adi Mantra three or more times.

Ong

Namo

Guru

Dev

Namo

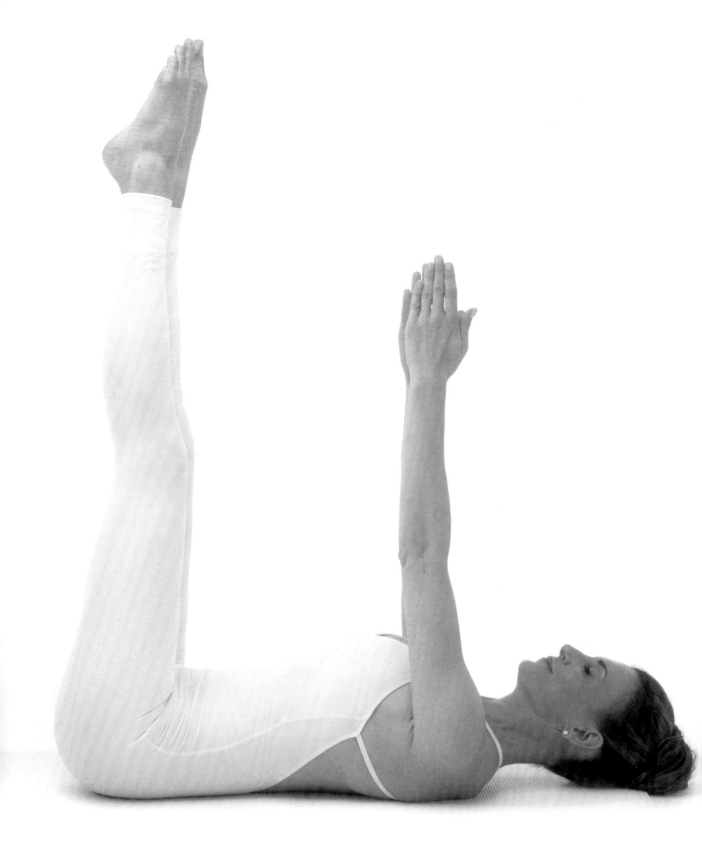

○ 2 TRUE U

1   Lie down, keeping your back pressed against the floor.
Lift your legs and arms straight up toward the sky, with
knees and elbows straight, toes and fingers pointed up.

2   Take very long, slow breaths deeply into your abdomen.
Hold the position for three to eleven minutes while
breathing. (Note that whatever amount of time you
choose, it will stay the same for the next three exercises
as well.) Feel your breathing sustaining you as you hold
the pose. Feel the energetic connection between your
spine and the earth and between your hands and feet.

3   To finish, inhale deeply, hold your breath, and then release your
legs and arms down to the ground as you exhale. Lie on your
back and take the time to allow your circulation to come back
to normal. Stay connected with your breathing as you rest.

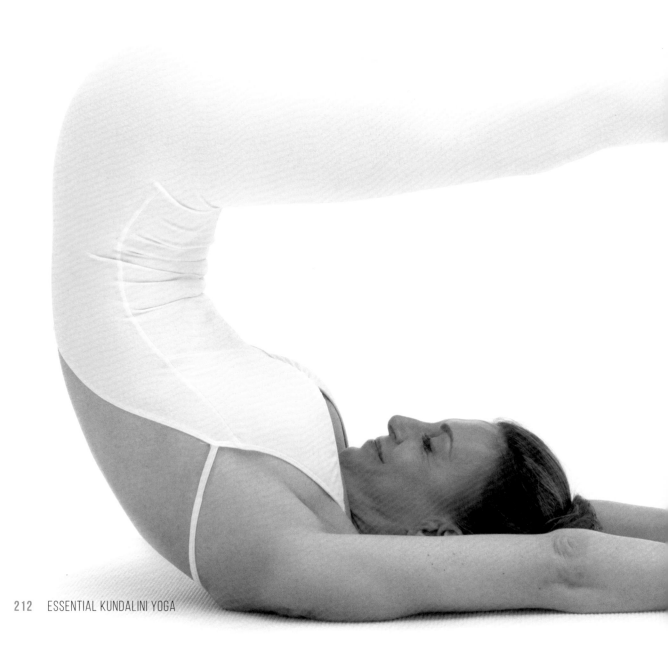

○ 3 GOT YOUR BACK U

1 While still lying on your back, stretch your arms over your head so they are flat on the ground. Raise your legs, pelvis, and lower spine up so your legs are pointing toward the sky. Then curl up your abdomen and lower your legs back over your head until they are parallel to the ground and to your arms.

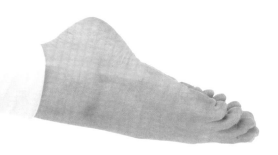

2 Hold the position and breathe slowly and deeply for the same amount of time as you held the previous pose, three to eleven minutes. Observe the flow of energy as you breathe.

3 To finish, exhale as you return your legs and arms to your starting position on your back. Take time to relax and assimilate the energies stimulated by these exercises so far.

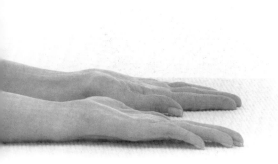

○ 4 ROW BOAT U

1 Sit up tall on the floor with your legs stretched out in front of you. Allow your spine to rise up perpendicular to the floor. Keeping the spine steady, elongate it and open the spaces between the vertebrae from the pelvis to the top of your head.

2 Reach your arms straight out in front of you, extending your fingers away from the shoulders. Hold this position and breathe deeply into your abdomen for the same amount of time as in the prior exercises, three to eleven minutes.

3 If you begin to feel uncomfortable, please remind yourself that you are readjusting your energy and then return your focus to the breath. This is a great time to recite a positive affirmation: "I am Light. I am Love. I am guided and protected. I am safe. All is well."

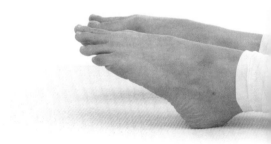

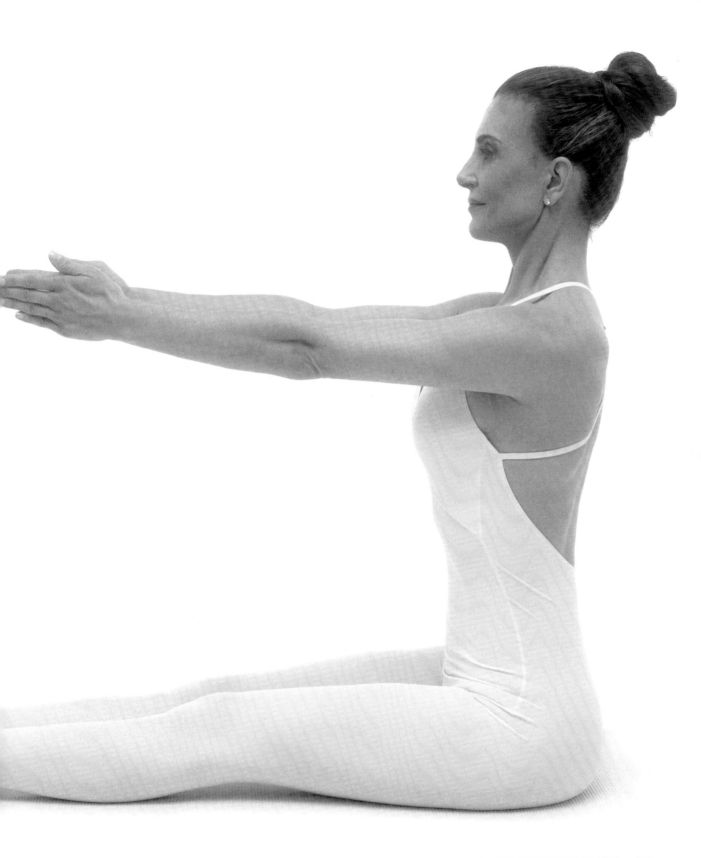

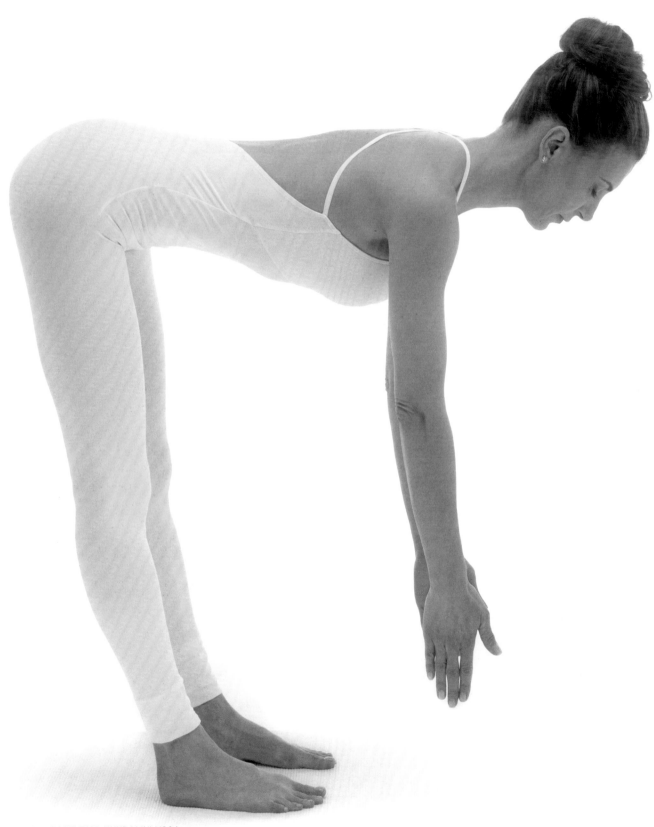

○ 5 INVERTED U

1   Stand up straight and tall. Plant your feet firmly on the ground shoulder width apart. Feel a line of energy rising up from the earth and extending through your spine, from your pelvis to the top of your head.

2   Bend forward from the hips until your torso is parallel to the ground. Keep your back parallel to the floor, legs straight, and buttocks high. Imagine that you are holding a tray with fragile cups of hot tea on your back. Allow your arms to dangle down with the fingers extended.

3   Hold this position and breathe with long, deep, aware, complete breaths. Feel the love in your breath circulating through your lungs, your heart, your energetic pathways, and your aura. Continue for the same amount of time you chose for the first three postures.

4   To finish, maintain the position and inhale and exhale deeply. At the end of the exhale, hold the breath out and pull Root Lock to consolidate your energy. Then inhale as you slowly rise up to standing, beginning the movement at your lower back and ascending one vertebra at a time. Again, take the time to feel yourself standing on the earth, with your spine straight and beautiful.

○ 6 DEEP RELAXATION

Immediately lie down on your back, cover yourself with a blanket made of wool or cotton, let your palms rest face up alongside your body, and relax deeply. We invite you to feel the waves of the universal energy washing through your electromagnetic field. Feel the love that the earth has for you and your connection with the angels. Allow and believe. Do not discount any feelings that arise. This is the time to trust and to allow the wisdom you've released to flow through your consciousness.

KRIYA FOR RADIANT SKIN

When we block our emotions, we dull our radiance, and this is reflected in dull, listless skin tone. The following set helps clear our subconscious mind so we can be free to show our natural brilliance to the world. The visible result is a wonderful natural glow. Allow yourself to get lost in the three motions and feel the joy in them. We are filled with energy when we recognize our calling is to love. This set is also excellent for toning the glutes, thighs, calves, and lower back.

○ 1 TUNE IN

Ong

Namo

Guru

Dev

Namo

1 Sit up in a cross-legged position and slow your breathing down, feeling it flowing deeply into your abdomen and your ribs, expanding them with each inhale.

2 When you are ready, bring your hands together in prayer position in front of your heart and chant the Adi Mantra three times or more.

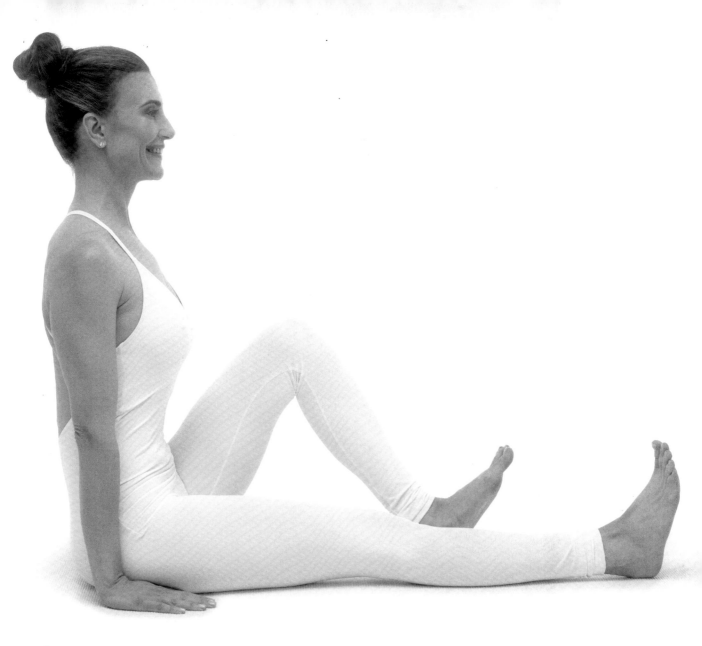

○ 2   SEATED KNEE LIFTS

1   Sit on the floor with your legs stretched out in front of you
and palms on the ground on either side of your hips. Begin
lifting alternate knees up and down, as though pedaling the
legs. Keep your heels on the ground, allowing them to slide
with the knee movement. You will soon feel an effect in your
thighs and abdomen, which will stimulate your glandular
system to release neuropeptides for cellular regeneration and
detoxification. Continue for thirty seconds to three minutes.

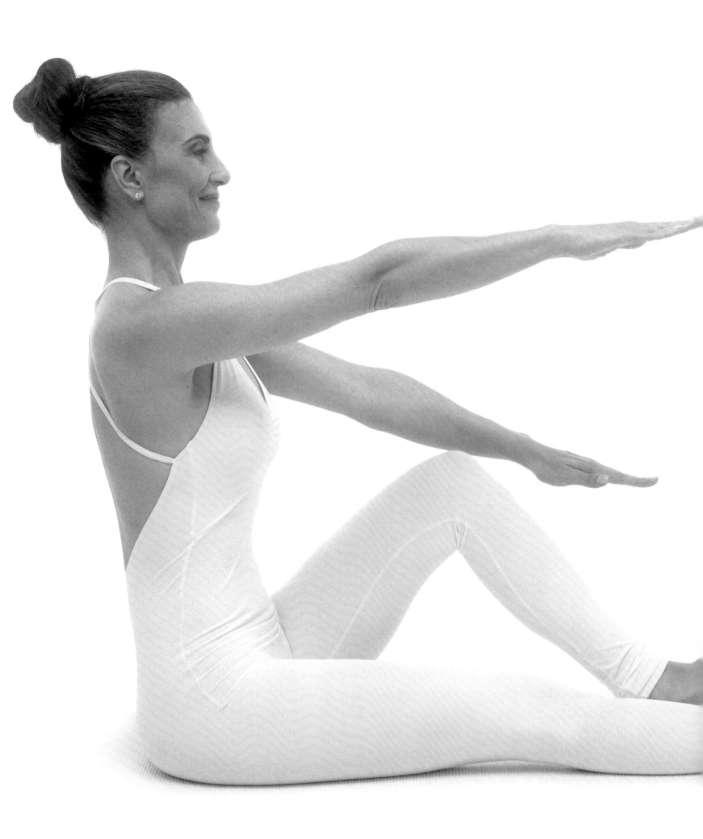

○ 3 SEATED KNEE AND ARM LIFTS

1 Keeping your legs moving with the same motion as in the previous exercise, extend your arms straight out in front of your shoulders and begin moving them up and down in rhythm with the legs. Get yourself going fast and lose yourself in the rhythm. Your pores may open and you may sweat, which is very healthy for releasing toxins.

2 Continue for two and a half to fifteen minutes. The motion will become meditative through its own movement. Focus on your breathing and relax into the movement.

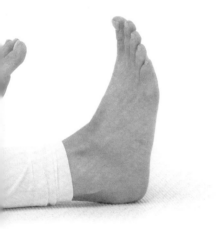

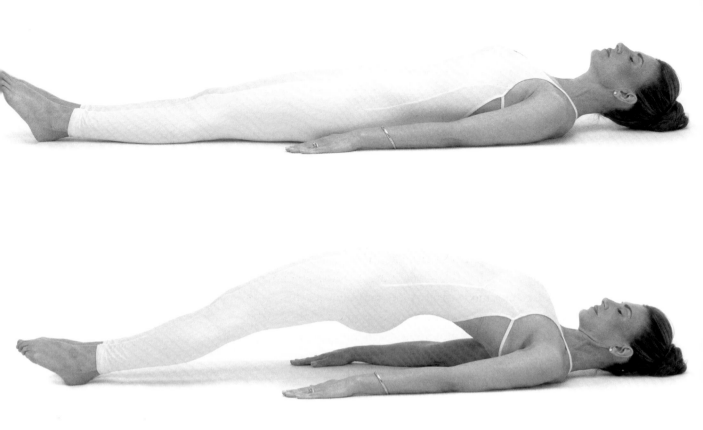

○ 4 JUMPING BEANS ON BACK

MODIFICATION Bend your knees and bring your heels closer to your buttocks. The closer your heels are, the easier it will be to lift your hips.

1 Lie down onto your back. Keeping your knees as straight as possible, lift the hips up and down, suspending your weight as an arch between the heels and the shoulders. Choose a rhythm that feels right for you. We suggest you inhale as your hips come up and exhale as they come down.

2 Move more quickly as your spine warms up. Continue for one and a half to fifteen minutes.

3 To finish, inhale in the up position, hold the breath as long as comfortably possible, and apply Root Lock. Exhale and relax down onto your back.

○ 5 JUMPING BEANS ON BELLY

Turn over so you are lying on your stomach. Lift your hips up and down by flexing and releasing the lower spine. Continue bouncing the hips up and down quickly for two to thirteen minutes. This motion stimulates the second chakra so that your energy can be strong, bright, and delightful.

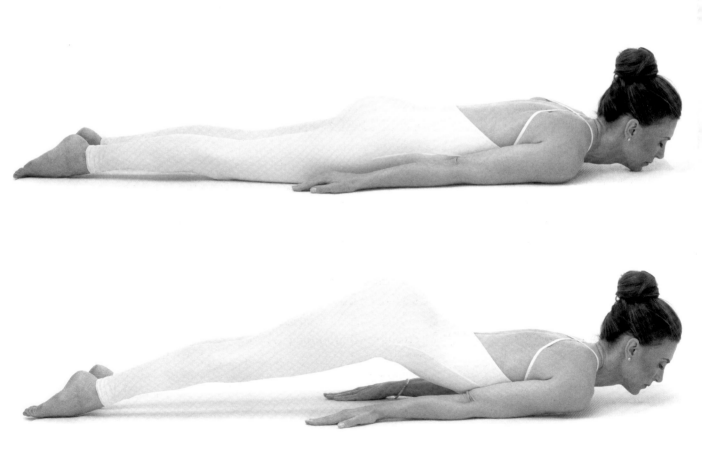

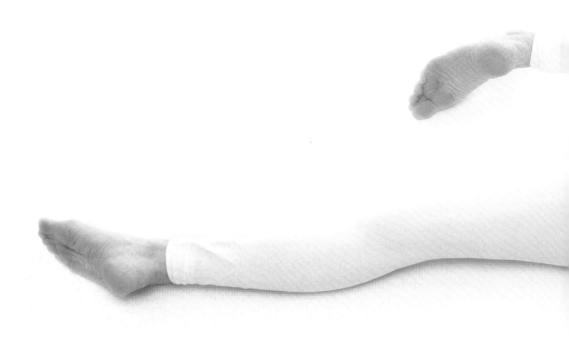

○ 6 CAT STRETCH

1 Lie on your back with your legs straight. Bend your left knee, hug it in toward your chest, and cross it over your torso toward the ground on the right side of your body. Your right buttock will lift off the ground, and your back will twist to the right. At the same time turn your head to the right and keep your shoulders as flat on the ground as possible.

2 Change sides, twisting the left bent knee over the straight right leg, turning the head to the left, and keeping your shoulders on the ground as much as possible.

3 Continue twisting from side to side this way for up to four minutes.

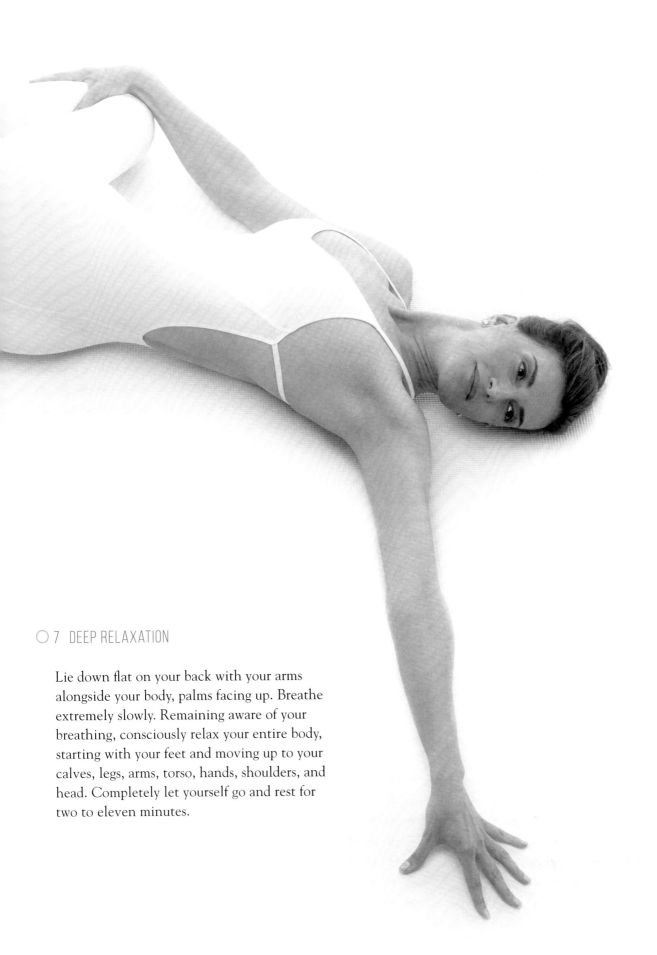

○ 7 DEEP RELAXATION

Lie down flat on your back with your arms alongside your body, palms facing up. Breathe extremely slowly. Remaining aware of your breathing, consciously relax your entire body, starting with your feet and moving up to your calves, legs, arms, torso, hands, shoulders, and head. Completely let yourself go and rest for two to eleven minutes.

STRENGTHENING THE AURA TO ATTRACT

When we clear the aura of density, the light of our soul vibrates with our truth and attracts our soul-level desires. Our frequency becomes so uplifted that our aura does the work for us, and what we project outward is attracted to us easily and divinely.

Sometimes people walk around with a flashlight looking for a gem on the ground, not realizing that the gem has been within them the entire time. We do not need to do anything except set our vibration free to shine so the infinite can draw things to us. An acorn becomes a tree, a seed grows into a flower, embryos become babies, and babies learn to walk. These are all spiritual doings, and either we choose to be part of that process or we are resistant to it.

When we truly embrace the beauty that resides within us and around us, we become a magnet for miracles, and we recognize that what we are searching for is already close by. If we understand the science of clearing the aura, we find we are able to surrender and relax in our day-to-day existence. If, on the other hand, we push for control, we can cut off the potential for cocreating with the wisdom of the universe. By allowing our light to shine, we permit the universe to clear a path for our soul, and our entire life changes.

○ 1 STANDING TUNE IN

Ong
Namo
Guru
Dev
Namo

1 Stand up tall with your legs shoulder width apart, feeling your weight evenly balanced on both feet, your spine rising from your pelvis to the top of your head, and the flow of breath entering and exiting your lungs. Sense how the energetic vibration of you extends into the space around your body and how the space comes into your body as well.

2 When you are ready, chant the Adi Mantra.

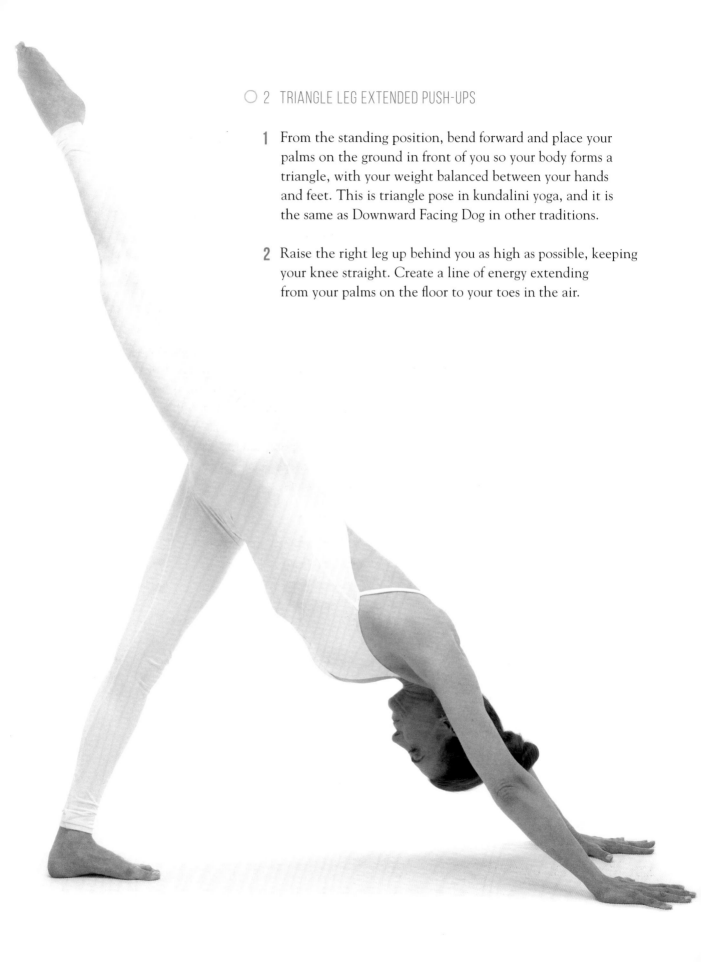

2 TRIANGLE LEG EXTENDED PUSH-UPS

1 From the standing position, bend forward and place your palms on the ground in front of you so your body forms a triangle, with your weight balanced between your hands and feet. This is triangle pose in kundalini yoga, and it is the same as Downward Facing Dog in other traditions.

2 Raise the right leg up behind you as high as possible, keeping your knee straight. Create a line of energy extending from your palms on the floor to your toes in the air.

3 With the right leg raised, exhale, bend the arms, and bring the forehead close to the ground. Inhale, straighten your arms, and rise up to the original Downward Facing Dog pose as described in step 1. Continue push-ups with the right leg raised for one and a half minutes.

4 To finish, inhale deeply, extend the leg and arms tall, and hold for a moment. Then bring your knees down and relax down out of the position.

5 Switch legs and do the raise-legged push-ups for another one and a half minutes. This exercise strengthens the arms tremendously, and it extends the power of projection and protection from the light body.

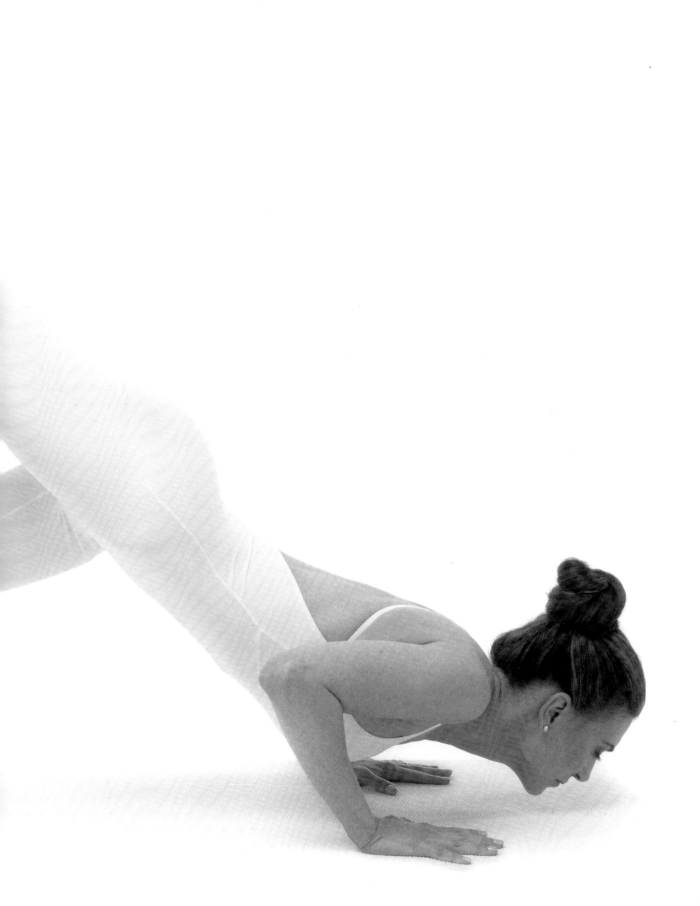

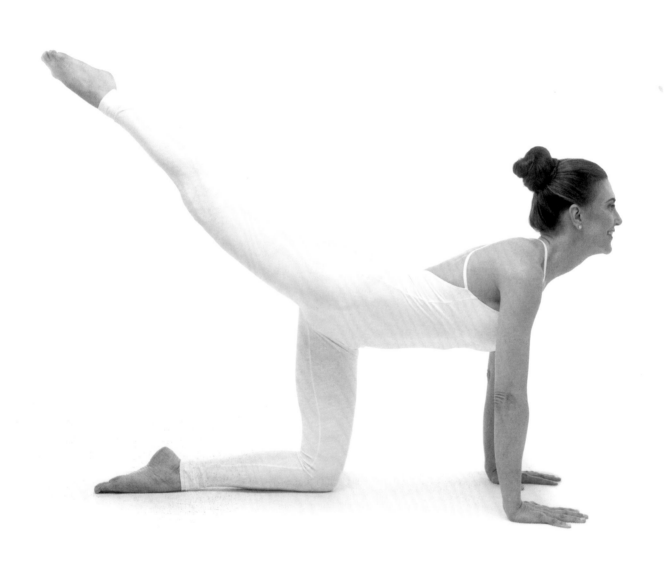

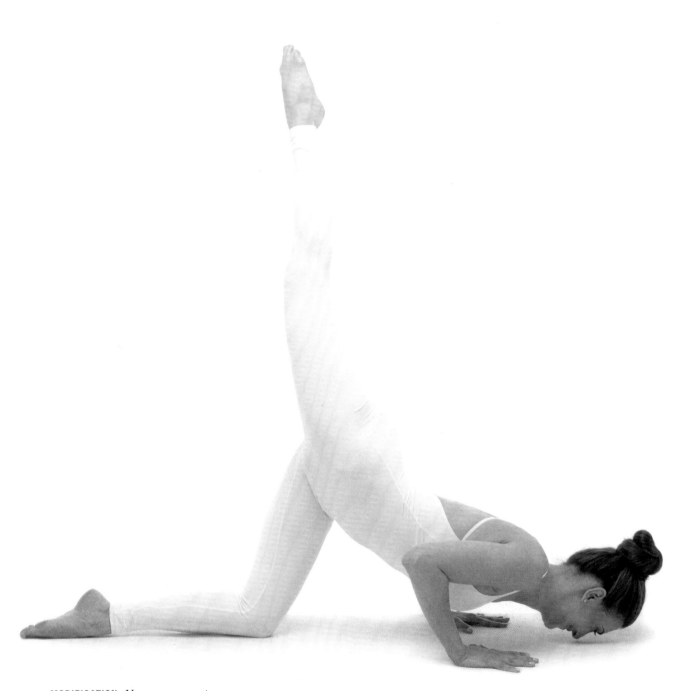

MODIFICATION You can practice this on your hands and knees while lifting the leg only as high as you can behind you.

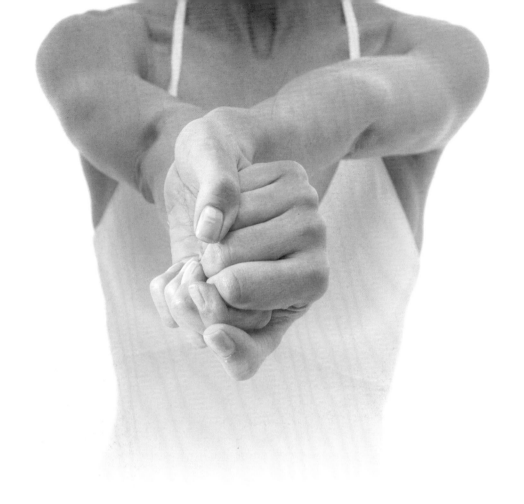

○ 3 ARM PUMP

1 Sit up in a cross-legged position with your spine straight.
Extend your left hand forward with the palm facing right,
as if you are about to grasp a pole. With the palm down, cross
your right hand under your left wrist and then lay the right
palm against the back of the left hand. Grasp the back of
the left hand by wrapping your right fingers over the top
of it. Both palms should face right. Extend your arms straight
out from your shoulders and keep your elbows locked.

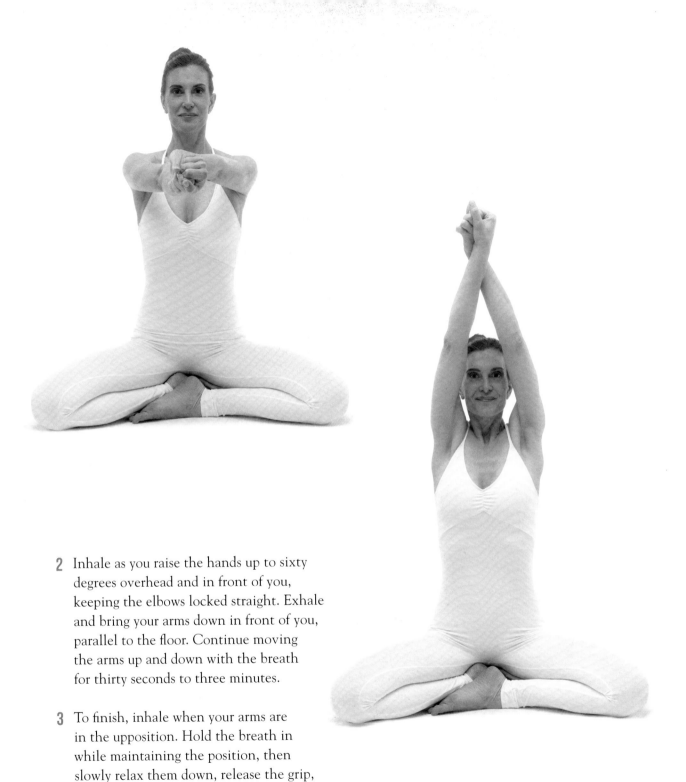

2 Inhale as you raise the hands up to sixty
   degrees overhead and in front of you,
   keeping the elbows locked straight. Exhale
   and bring your arms down in front of you,
   parallel to the floor. Continue moving
   the arms up and down with the breath
   for thirty seconds to three minutes.

3 To finish, inhale when your arms are
   in the upposition. Hold the breath in
   while maintaining the position, then
   slowly relax them down, release the grip,
   and transition to normal breathing.

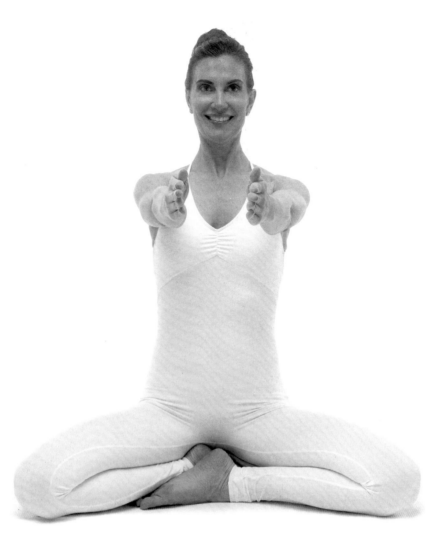

○ 4 ARM SWING

1 Stay seated upright with your legs crossed. Stretch both arms out in front of you, parallel to the ground, with elbows straight. Have your palms facing each other six inches apart.

2 As you inhale, swing your arms wide apart to either side and behind you. As you exhale, bring them back to the original position. As you repeat the same action, we invite you to imagine that a powerful light is coming through your fingertips and you are combing through your energy field, clearing any old or stuck energy that does not serve you. Feel that you are protecting your energy field from heavy or dense energy that wants to stick to you. Continue this back-and-forth arm motion for one to three minutes.

3 To finish, inhale deeply with the arms open and then exhale as you relax the arms down.

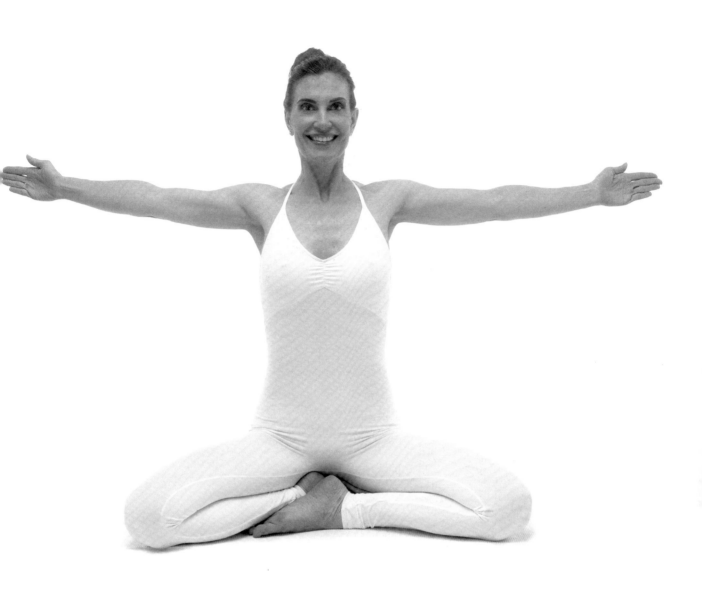

○ 5 DEEP RELAXATION

Relax on your back and allow your physical and energetic body
to assimilate the practice. Feel the glow around you as it heals
any leftover stuck energy that needs to dissolve. This is the most
important part of the exercise. Continue to focus on the golden
glow around you—you are like a shining sun projecting rays of
light in all directions. Be still and know you are manifesting your
dreams as you rest.

DETOXING FOR RADIANCE

When our digestion is clear and healthy, it is reflected in our complexion and our radiance. The following set of exercises is amazing for the tummy. It balances the intestinal flora and aids digestion. It helps to prevent depression by eliminating unhealthy bacteria and clearing old toxins. It works wonders for losing weight. This is a great set to practice if you have stomach issues or are taking antibiotics. It gives energy to our radiance. The set uses Venus Lock which is explained in chapter 7.

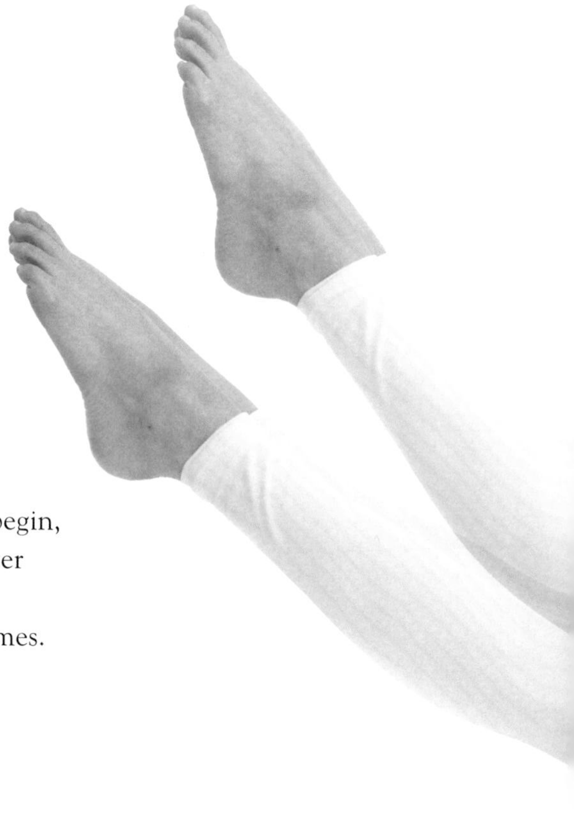

○ 1 TUNE IN

Ong

Namo

Guru

Dev

Namo

1 Sit up in a cross-legged position. Slow your breathing down, feeling it flowing deeply into your abdomen and your ribs, expanding them with each inhale.

2 When you are ready to begin, place your hands in prayer pose and chant the Adi Mantra three or more times.

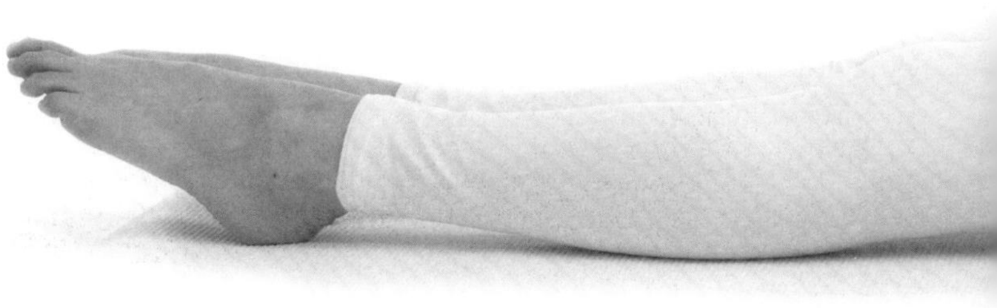

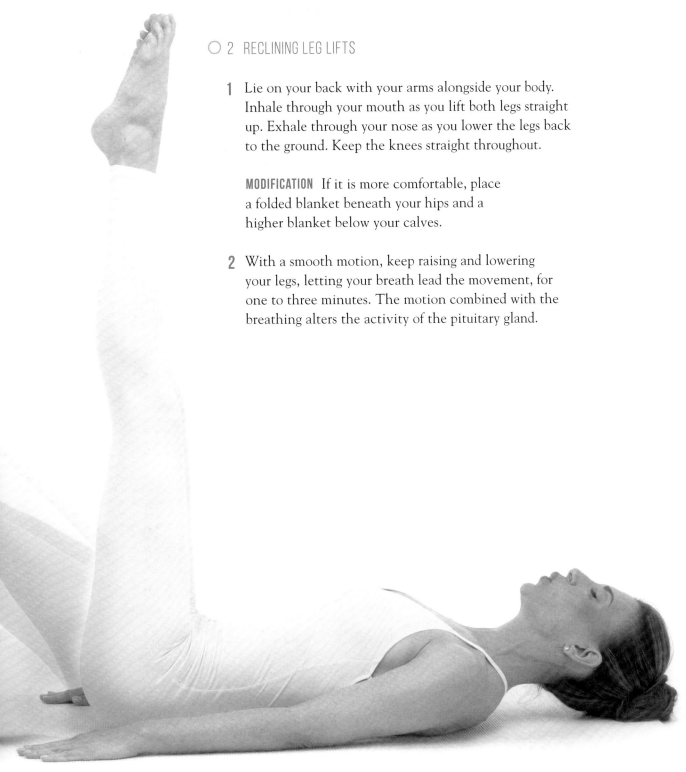

○ 2   RECLINING LEG LIFTS

1   Lie on your back with your arms alongside your body.
Inhale through your mouth as you lift both legs straight
up. Exhale through your nose as you lower the legs back
to the ground. Keep the knees straight throughout.

MODIFICATION   If it is more comfortable, place
a folded blanket beneath your hips and a
higher blanket below your calves.

2   With a smooth motion, keep raising and lowering
your legs, letting your breath lead the movement, for
one to three minutes. The motion combined with the
breathing alters the activity of the pituitary gland.

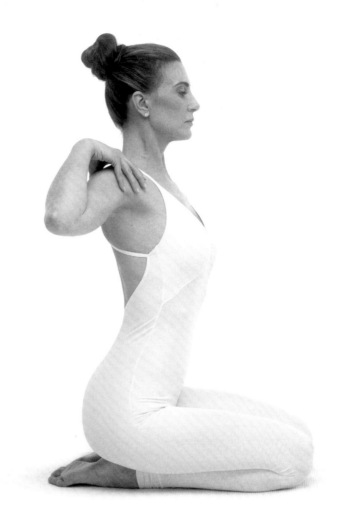

○ 3 ROCK POSE TO KNEELING

1 Immediately after completing the leg lifts, sit on your
heels in Rock Pose, with your hands on your shoulders.

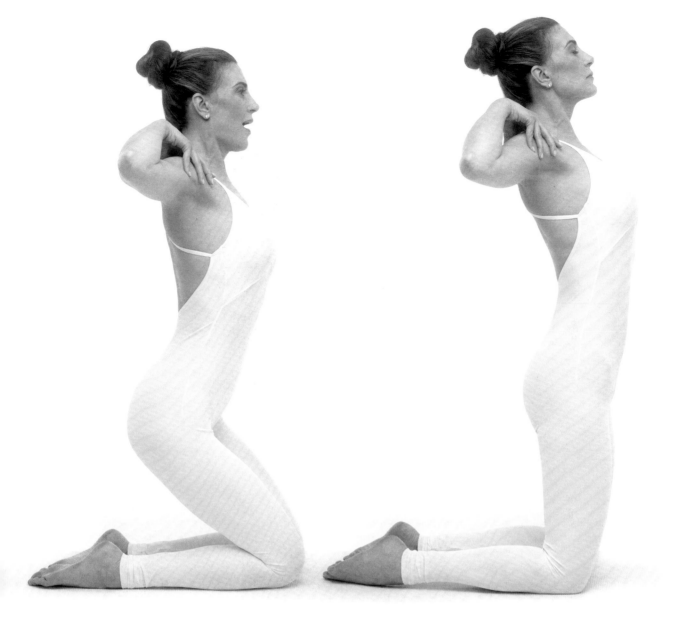

2 Inhale through your mouth and lift your hips up so you are in a kneeling position. As you come up, bring your hips forward and your elbows back, straightening the spine. Keep the head level and facing forward.

3 Exhale through your nose and return to the original starting position.

4 Continue the up-and-down motion and accompanying breath pattern vigorously for one to three and a half minutes. Increase the pace as you warm up.

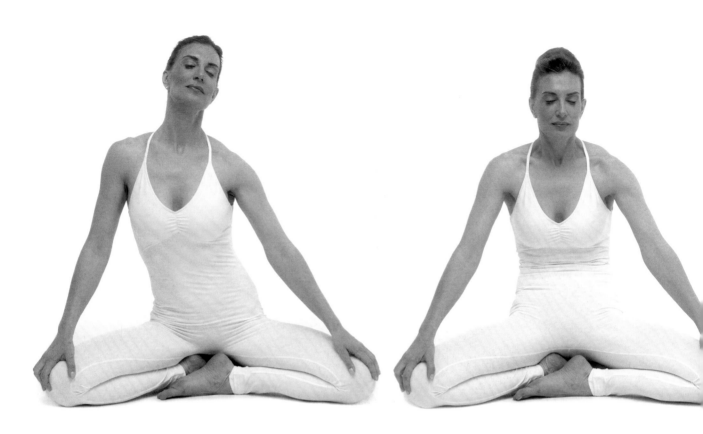

○ 4 THE DIVINE GRIND

1 Sit down in a cross-legged position. Place your hands on your
knees. Begin to churn your lower torso, making big circles
by moving your navel to the front, side, back, opposite side,
and front again. Allow your chin to come up naturally as you
churn your spine forward and down as you churn backward.
Coordinate the movement with your breath by inhaling as
you rotate your torso forward and exhaling as you arc it back.

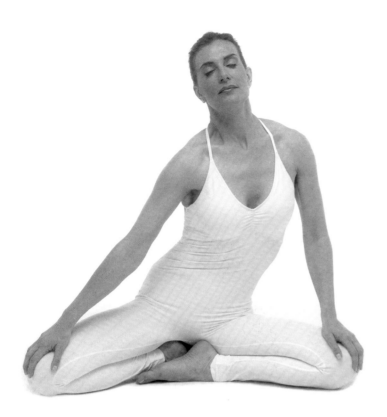

2 Continue for one to three and a half minutes. We suggest reversing the direction halfway through. This motion aids in digestion and helps remove toxins from the kidneys, gallbladder, liver, and spleen. It also balances the adrenal glands.

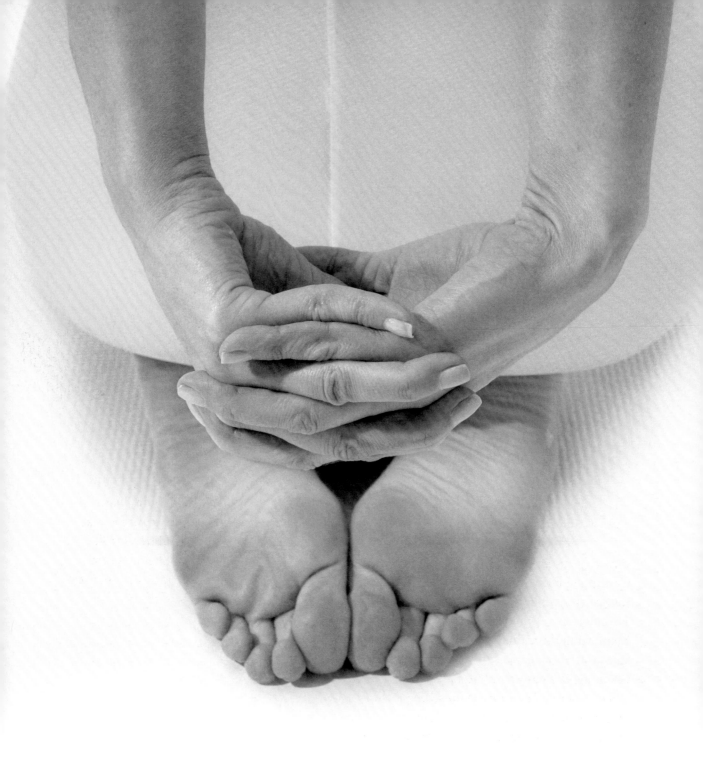

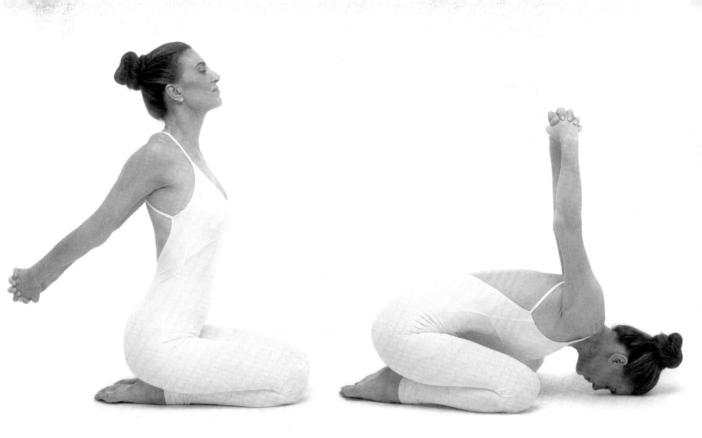

○ 5 ACTIVE YOGA MUDRA

1 Sit up tall in Easy Pose. Interlock your hands behind
   you in Venus Lock, with the fingers interlaced.

2 Inhaling through the mouth, lower your forehead
   toward the floor in front of you while lifting the
   folded hands as high as possible behind you.

3 Rise back up straight and tall as you exhale through the nose.

4 Continue the movement and breathe for one to
   three minutes. The unusual breathing technique of
   inhaling on the forward bend will give a beneficial
   massage to the intestines and abdominal organs.

MODIFICATION Sit on your
heels, as pictured. You may
find it helpful to straddle
a folded blanket or a firm
cushion by placing it between
your heels to sit on.

○ 6 RELAXATION WITH NAVEL FOCUS

1 Lie down on your back and bring your focus to your navel point, mentally directing your prana to the energy center there. The navel point is an essential part of your awakening. It is the power center of your consciousness. As you focus, relax with your palms face up alongside your body.

2 Slow down your breath, relax every fiber of your body, and visualize your body melting into the earth's gravity. Feel the light of the universe washing through your aura. Scan your entire body, from your feet to your head, and consciously relax every muscle. Continue resting for five to seven minutes.

PART 3

THE FIELD OF POSSIBILITIES

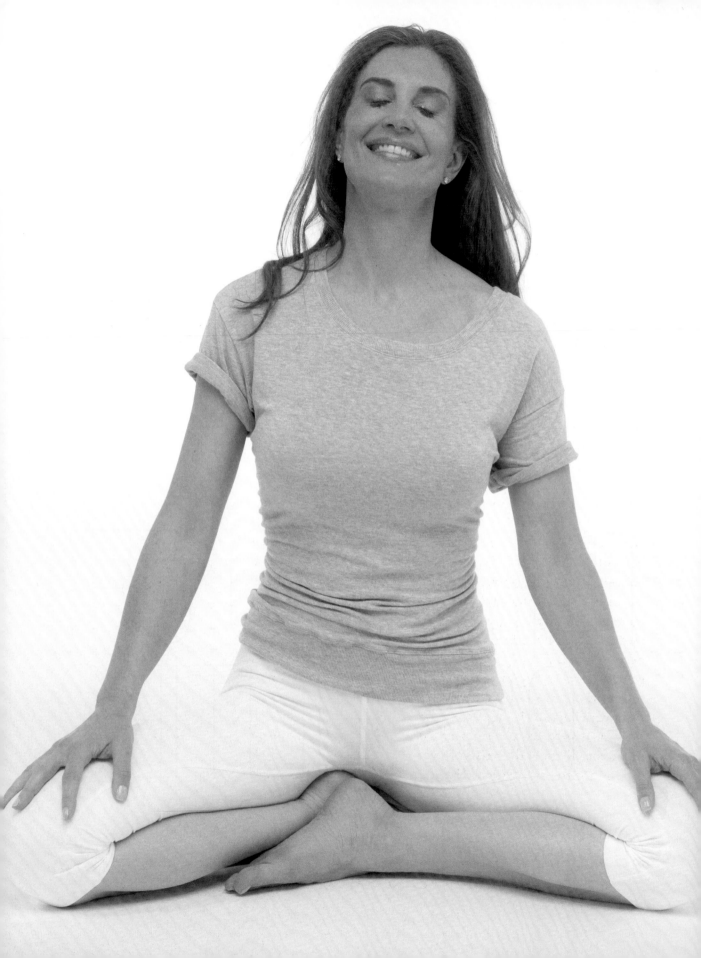

9 NATURALLY ATTRACTIVE ENERGY

Darkness cannot drive out darkness; only light can do that.
MARTIN LUTHER KING JR.

WE HAVE THE POTENTIAL TO sparkle and shine in ways that we may not even be aware of. The electromagnetic field around our body is an activation field—a vortex of potential that draws in what it resonates with. We live within a universe of infinite possibilities, but our limited beliefs and self-concepts often hold us back from expanding to our fullest potential. Within this field we hold many resonant imprints—some that work wonders but many that no longer serve us. Subconscious imprints from our family's beliefs and from our own experiences remain as opaque blocks to our radiance. Once we let go of the limiting beliefs, however, our lives can expand and flow in seemingly miraculous ways.

By purifying our electromagnetic field of resistances, we can align with and draw in our deepest heart's desires. This purification is an activation. Without the resistance we've been carrying, our true self can shine without distortion. The power of this activation is one of the greatest gifts you can take from this book. By tapping into the activation field—the magnetic field of your aura—you can create a life of peace, joy, and fulfillment.

DESIRE

Don't go and get it; be and allow it to come to you.
YOGI BHAJAN

Desire is a beautiful emotion that can allow us to recognize that the universe is working through us. Desire and want are very different. Lust is a want; desire is of the soul. Wanting comes from the mindset of lack and fear. Desire comes from the heartfelt longing to fulfill a divine purpose. One repels, and the other attracts. Wanting creates a field of resistance. Desire works in alignment with the divine. Many people are confused about the law of attraction because they are setting intentions based on wanting instead of on desiring, not realizing they are two quite different energies.

Desire emits a high frequency in which our resonance aligns with the universe, signaling that we are ready, and the universe is ready as well. When the energy comes from the soul's passionate inspiration, we have an ability to surrender with detachment, knowing that what we desire from the heart is on its way. The problem with wanting is that it is an attachment that comes from the ego. We have an innate drive to be successful, but people sometimes strive and push so hard to make things happen that they actually block the chance for the infinite wisdom of the universe to fulfill their desire in ways they never imagined. Divine desire is for the highest good of all and can never hurt another person.

We are all born with a destiny, and that destiny calls to us with a feeling of heartfelt desire. When our desire is of the heart and soul, the universe assists us, because by pursuing a calling we are invoking the very force that God gave us in the first place. The sensation of desire that arises from your calling is a stimulus to action coming from the divine.

When we live and serve from the heart, desire becomes something we trust God has planted within us. Dreams do come true. When we live from the heart and clarify our intention, the universe takes care of all of our needs in the proper time.

By releasing our attachment to an outcome, we allow it to arrive. We vibrate with the trust that we are divine vessels, following the guidance that flows through our hearts as we accomplish the tasks before us. This way we allow God to work through us. We do our work with love, and then more love arrives. It is a cycle. God is the doer. Surrendering the ego and laying the soul on the vast grasses of the meadow under the clouds and sunshine of God's love will open the field of possibilities.

By tapping into the activation field— the electromagnetic field of your aura—you cause things to start moving. The secret is to sit and vibrate rather than rushing around pursuing goals. Feel the result as having being achieved. Feel every sensation. Feel the gratitude for your success as a physical sensation within your body. The following exercise and visualization will create the vibration within your electromagnetic field that aligns the divine and your desire at a soul level.

○ PATIENCE PAYS AFFIRMATION

When we do not know what our destiny is and we feel confused, impatient, or doubtful, we remember the dreams we had as children and recognize that usually our greatest childhood joys are part of the divine plan.

1 Sit on the floor with your legs out straight in front of you. Connect with your breathing, paying attention to the inhale and the exhale.

2 Close your eyes and bend forward, folding over your straight legs so you are in a position of surrender. This posture is called Seated Forward Bend. It is the yoga

pose of pure surrender. Folding forward allows the heart
to lead the way so the mind can follow the love.

3   Breathe deeply and repeat aloud the words: "Patience pays. Let
the hand of God work for me." Continue for three minutes.

4   Observe the relaxation that occurs within you and around you.
It is like a miracle. And it is more real than anything you
see with your physical eyes. You are so very loved.

GRATITUDE ATTRACTS

Gratitude is the open door to abundance.
YOGI BHAJAN

The vibration we feel as gratitude sends waves of positive energy
through our body, our aura, and the external circles of our life. By
consciously directing our attention to whatever we are grateful for
and allowing that feeling to resonate in our body, we establish a clear
vibration within our electromagnetic field that echoes with those
potentials in the external world. This is the law of sympathetic resonance. When we focus on feelings of thankfulness, we create space
for the arrival of more things to be grateful for. By adding sound, in
the form of a mantra, to that vibration, we amplify the effect as the
sound carries the gratitude frequency into the physical world.

Everyone faces challenges in life. It is part of being human. This
earth realm is the school for our soul, where we learn and grow
through our experiences. Oftentimes we are asked to recognize the
opportunities that arise from the challenges—to see the silver lining.
This can be incredibly difficult to do, just as it sometimes takes time
for a rainbow to appear after a storm. However, gratitude is one of
the most effective ways to move out of the lower frequencies that
come from fear, sadness, and anxiety.

Making gratitude a regular practice opens up the synaptic pathways inside our brain, so that gratitude becomes a go-to emotion in

times of difficulty. When we feel stuck and are finding it hard to be thankful, having a regular gratitude practice already in place can help immensely. We can begin by relishing every blessing we have in our lives and writing them all down. Waking in the morning to remember the many blessings you enjoy is a wonderful practice. And the vibration this habit creates in our attraction field draws more goodness into our lives.

"WAHE GURU" MEDITATION FOR GRATITUDE AND ECSTASY

Gratitude is our natural mind-set when we are connected to the divine. In the conscious practice of gratitude described below, we connect our inner intention with sound and meditative awareness using the mantra "Wahe Guru" (pronounced "*wah*-hay *guh*-roo"). Yogi Bhajan put it this way: "'Wahe Guru' is the inherent thank-you for all there is that brings us closer to light." This ancient mantra means "Ecstasy is here and now. Everything that was dark is now full of light."

Wahe Guru

If you do this as a practice for forty days, you will create a fertile space for more blessings to arrive.

1 Lie down on your back and relax completely. Close your eyes and begin to mentally list all the things you are grateful for.

2 Each time you think of something to be thankful for, say the mantra "Wahe Guru" out loud. This affirmation becomes a meditation, vibrating the thought into the physical realm using sound. As the sound infuses the world around you, it will carry the vibration of gratitude into all the matter within you and surrounding you—your body, the walls, the air.

○ THE ADVANCE GRATITUDE TECHNIQUE

The Advance Gratitude Technique is an exercise that we developed together while teaching a few years ago.

The Advance Gratitude Technique uses our energetic body to vibrate into the potential of the physical world. It brings amazing results and can only be used for good. The four steps—relaxing, envisioning, sensing, and cultivating—build on and work in harmony with one another to create a coherent energy. As we continue to practice, we simply get better at it, and the results compound into a miraculous state of being.

Once you have spent time listening inside, clearing your vibration, and activating your light with the exercises in this book, simply allow yourself to trust that what you desire is also calling to you and is on its way.

1 **RELAX COMPLETELY** The first step is to sit where you can be comfortable or lie down on your back. Following the relaxation techniques previously described in this book, take long, slow, and deep breaths. Focus completely on your breathing. Relax every muscle in your body. Allow your jaw to drop slightly open. Just breathe. By relaxing, you are activating your parasympathetic nervous system and allowing your inner glow to project beyond your physical body, becoming an outer glow expanding into your aura. Continue for one to five minutes.

2 **ENVISION** The next step is to clearly envision your most heartfelt desire. Create a strong, coherent picture in your mind. We have two physical eyes for outer sight and we have a third eye for insight. Give yourself permission to truly see what you wish for with all of your eyes. Notice every detail. Do not judge. Do not think anything is impossible. The only task is to clearly picture what you desire.

Envision that what you are attracted to is good for all those you are in relationship with and good for your own well-being. Trust that there is a sacred reason you are desiring it. As mentioned earlier, spirit speaks to us through our high-frequency desires.

Permit yourself the pleasure of the possibility. Allow that whatever the universe is drawing you toward is for the highest good of all. Trust the goodness of your own soul. *Visualize. Visualize. Visualize.* As we stated earlier, by tapping into the activation field—the electromagnetic field of our aura—we start things moving.

3 EXPLORE PHYSICAL SENSATION The third step is to create the sensation within your physical body of already having what you have envisioned, right here and now. Explore the feeling in every detail, allowing it to enter and fill your body as though the desire has already been fulfilled. Feel it very tangibly and physically as a distinct sensation in your muscles, bones, and heart. See it, smell it, taste it, hear it.

Deeply immerse yourself in the pleasurable sensation of having what you desire. Allow that enjoyment to ripple though you and stay with it. For many this can feel sensual. For some their skin tingles. You may feel a wonderful physical sensation in your back, your ribs, or your abdomen. Your dream is here right now.

4 EXPERIENCE GRATITUDE The fourth step is to cultivate immense gratitude for that very feeling inside. It is essential to feel the gratitude for this beautiful inner sensation you are having right now rather than for the abstract, external idea. It is a sensation of immense satisfaction and bliss. Give thanks from your mind to your heart and from your heart to your energy field. The desire you envision as fulfilled is real. It is possible. It is beautiful. Say aloud three times: "Thank you. Thank you. Thank you."

When we give thanks in advance for our most heartfelt dreams, we create a dynamic of readiness. Your electromagnetic field becomes a highly attractive force. You establish yourself as a radiant being blossoming from fertile ground to receive the miracles that are on their way. The wonders of the universe are so very obtainable when you activate them with gratitude.

10 UNLOCKING ENERGETIC DOORWAYS

*It is not the magnitude of our actions but the amount
of love that is put into them that matters.*
MOTHER TERESA

IN THIS CHAPTER WE EXPLORE a number of profound ways to utilize the power of kundalini yoga to transform our lives. Yoga opens the gateway for energy to move, and as the gateway opens, our enhanced energy begins flowing into all the corners of our life.

We discuss challenges that are common to humanity in this modern age and offer practices that help shift our energy so we can be as amazing as we have the potential to be. Something extraordinary happens when we see the gifts that come from pressure. Just as pressurized carbon becomes a diamond, our lives can sparkle when we expand away from the low vibratory contractions of shame, fear, guilt, anger, and sorrow.

FOCUS

Our ability to focus depends on our inner capability to concentrate prana. When the movement of prana within our brain is restricted and scattered, our cognitive functioning becomes restricted and scattered as well. In this era of advanced technology, with distractions at every turn, many people find they have trouble focusing for even a short period of time. Yet the conduction of prana through the brain can be powerfully enhanced with an ancient technique known as *Kirtan Kriya.*

This meditation is one of the most highly studied yoga practices of the modern era. Scientists at the University of California, Los Angeles, reported in a 2016 double-blind study that subjects who practiced Kirtan Kriya improved cognitive function, boosted memory, and increased blood flow to their brains. Numerous other studies have shown similar findings. While its effects have been scientifically verified, this age old yogic meditation is also easy enough for everyone.

○ KIRTAN KRIYA

This technique combines four unique elements: an ancient mantra, a phased way of chanting, a finger movement, and a visualization.

MANTRA

Saa
Taa
Naa
Maa

The mantra consists of four simple syllables that were revered by the sages and have been used for meditation over millennia: "Saa," "Taa," "Naa," and "Maa." *Saa* means "infinity," *Taa* means "incarnation," *Naa* means "transformation," and *Maa* means "regeneration." You do not have to know or contemplate the meanings, however, in order to do the meditation, since each syllable reverberates internally as pure sound to activate the flow of energy within the brain.

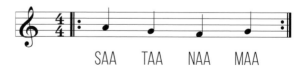

SAA   TAA   NAA   MAA

PHASED CHANTING

The mantra is chanted in six phases of equal duration. In the first phase the mantra is chanted out loud. In the second phase the mantra is whispered. In the third and fourth phases the mantra is vibrated silently. In the fifth phase the mantra is whispered, and in the sixth, it is chanted out loud again.

Before you begin, decide on the duration you want for the phases and have a timer or a clock ready. Each phase can span from one to thirty-one minutes, but take into account that the total practice time will end up being six times longer than a single phase. Each of the phases are equal in length. We recommend phases of two minutes or more to start.

FINGER MOVEMENT

Simply press your thumb to each of your fingertips in succession at the same time as you chant each syllable, as per the instructions in the steps below. The delicate stimulation of each fingertip coordinates the hemispheres of the brain and trains our mind to stay steadily in focus.

L-FORM VISUALIZATION

Kirtan Kriya employs a visualization of an L-shaped movement of sound. Imagine each syllable as a glistening orb of sound starting overhead, then entering through the fontanel, making a right turn in your midbrain, and exiting forward through the third eye point. The sound starts from infinity, passes through the finite self, and is released into infinity.

1   Begin by sitting up straight with your eyes closed and hands resting with the palms face up on your knees. Close your eyes and focus internally at your third eye. Take time to observe the flow of prana with every breath. Chant the Adi Mantra.

2   Say the syllable "Saa" out loud, while at the same time pressing the tips of your thumbs and index fingers together, as in Gyan Mudra. Visualize the sound as a vibrating orb that starts above

Ong

Namo

Guru

Dev

Namo

Saa

Taa

Naa

Maa

your head, drops down through the crown of your skull, vibrates through your midbrain, and exits directly forward through the third eye at the brow point, making the shape of an L.

3 As you say the second syllable, "Taa," press your thumbs against the tips of your middle fingers. Again visualize the sound as a vibration that enters through your fontanel, makes an L inside at the center of your head, and smoothly exits through your third eye.

4 As you say the third syllable, "Naa," press your thumbs to the tips of your ring fingers. Again visualize the L-shaped pathway of vibration as you did for the previous two syllables.

5 As you say the final syllable, "Maa," press your thumbs to the tip of your pinkies and visualize the sound entering your brain and exiting via the L-shaped pathway through your third eye.

6 Keep chanting the syllables one after the other at a steady, even pace, with the accompanying finger gestures. Each repetition of the entire four-syllable mantra should take about three seconds.

Without breaking the steady rhythm, briefly inhale following each repetition of the full mantra, "Saa, Taa, Naa, Maa."

7 Continue chanting out loud for the phase duration that you had decided upon before starting.

8 Once the first phase duration is finished, enter the second phase by chanting the mantra in a whisper. Continue the chanting, finger movements, and visualization for the same amount of time as the first phase.

9 For the third and fourth phases, silently imagine the sound "Saa, Taa, Naa, Maa" while continuing the finger movements

and the visualization. Listen inside as though you could hear the sound. Continue for twice the duration of a single phase.

10 For the fifth phase, whisper the mantra out loud again, accompanied by the finger movements and visualization.

11 For the sixth phase, chant with a full voice again while continuing the finger movements and visualization.

12 To finish, inhale, hold your breath, and stretch your fingers out wide. Exhale and relax your fingers. Sit for some time to observe the clarity of your brain and the reduction of stress. Can you feel your vibration as a clear channel sending messages of love?

CLEARING EMOTIONS FROM THE PAST

You run after wealth, glory, and glamour, but [they] will run after you, providing you are an open channel.
YOGI BHAJAN

If we are feeling the need to heal pain from the past, we have to do it with love. When we sever cords before God does it for us, we are making a statement to the universe that we do not trust the divine flow. We have a misconception that we need to protect ourselves from toxic people by cutting them out of our lives. By cutting someone out of our lives energetically, we are playing around with the light; whatever we cut out without healing first will come back to us in another form. We must feel it, heal it, and then release it to the wind. What we are being called to do is to love. Sometimes we do need to move away quickly from harmful people. However, in horrific relationships, we are being challenged and reminded to love ourselves. If a toxic person is destroying your life, move away, but make sure you heal your heart so you do not attract a similar energy again. Once you heal yourself you will not need to cut the cords, because they will be cut for you. Remember that energy cannot be created or destroyed. Energy can be redistributed. Energy is an endless source, and when we infuse darkness with light, we heal ourselves.

There is a new age misconception that is confusing to many people. Setting boundaries and taking more time to indulge in ourselves is supposed to make our lives better? The reality is that we were born to give our love, and by holding it back from others, we isolate ourselves. We long to heal our planet and one another—this is a primal yearning that arises from the soul. True happiness comes from opening our hearts and giving love to others. Have you ever felt lonely while you were using all your energy on taking care of your own needs instead of others? We often see this happen with parents when their kids move away from home. Their giving does not have a natural place to go. The healing comes from continuing to be a mother and father to others and to our world. When we dismiss the energy of yearning entirely, because we think it is negative, we are simply locking that energy inside our body. Shifting our energy is the answer. The following meditation utilizes our breathing to bring about that shift.

○ BREATHING TO CLEAR EMOTIONS FROM THE PAST

This breathing exercise is especially beneficial when we are dealing with stressful relationships. It works on eliminating our fears, removing unsettling thoughts, and even releasing issues going back as far as our past ancestral lineage. We must change our energy patterns in order to heal, and when we nurture our family karmic patterns, we are literally healing our own energy effortlessly and without the pain of severing a connection.

1 Sit in a comfortable position on the floor or in a chair. Slow down your breathing and observe the flow of breath entering and exiting your lungs.

2 Bring your fingertips together in front of your heart so that the tips touch opposite fingers and the palms are spread far apart.

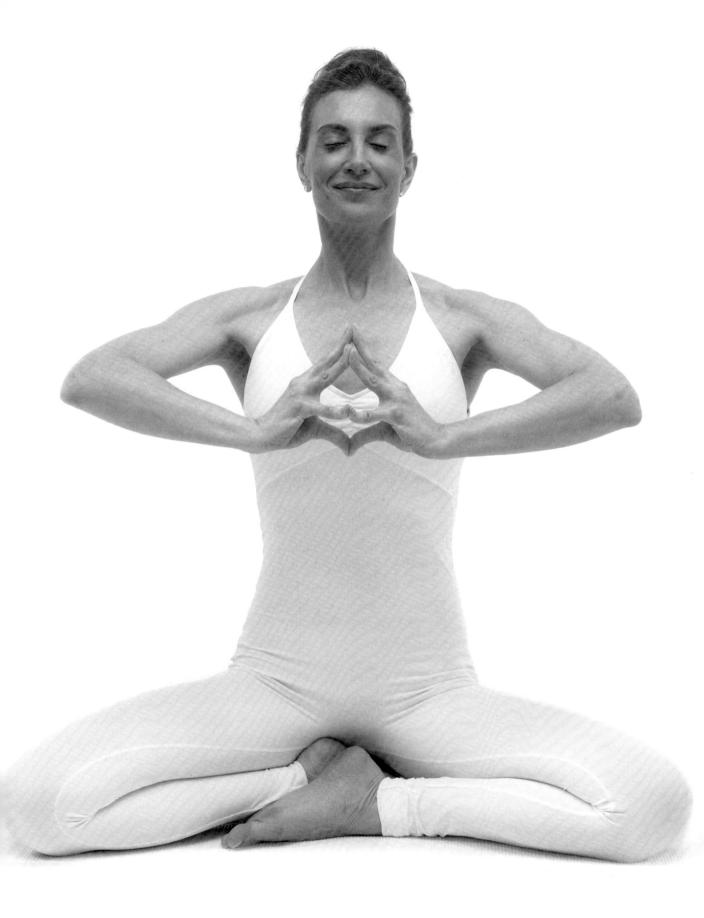

3 Lower your eyelids until they're almost closed, so that there is a small sliver of light coming in. Gaze at the very tip of your nose. This stabilizes the optic nerve and opens our intuition.

4 Using the Square Breath technique outlined in chapter 3, breathe as slowly as possible, inhaling for a count of eight, holding in for eight, exhaling for eight, and holding out for eight. Continue for eleven minutes, or until you feel a sense of relief from hurt feelings or other emotions that have been bothering you. Sometimes it will take only three minutes to shift out of the fear mind-set into the healing mind-set, where love takes over.

PROTECTIVE ENERGY SHIELD

Aad Guray Nameh
Jugaad Guray Nameh
Sat Guray Nameh
Siri Guru Davay Nameh

The arc line is a bright arc of energy in our electromagnetic field that radiates from ear to ear in the space over the hairline for men and women. Women have a second arc line that extends from nipple to nipple which is known to hold energetic wounds from past sexual relationships. A weak arc line allows negative energies to reach us, but when our arc line is vibrating with healthy divine energy, we have a shield of light protecting us.

The vibration of sound, such as mantra, is a very effective tool with which to charge our arc line and aura with a positive protective force. Mantras are so powerful they create a vibration that cancels out negative energies coming into our electromagnetic field. Imagine that you have a halo of light circling around your aura. The sound you create with these ancient mantras solidifies the circle. The vibrations themselves are making the halo strong and powerful. The mantras also heal past imprints that are stuck in the arc lines.

The mantra "Aad Guray Nameh, Jugaad Guray Nameh, Sat Guray Nameh, Siri Guru Davay Nameh" (pronounced "aad *guh-ray* na-meh, joo-*gaad* guh-*ray* na-meh, sutt guh-*ray* na-meh, *si*-ree guh-*roo day*-vay na-*meh*") is a profound sound vibration that fills our magnetic field with a protective light. As you chant, visualize four luminous columns of light that protect you on all four sides of your body. You create a safe zone inside these four protective lights. This mantra infuses our personal vibration with the protective energy that comes from perpetual timelessness. It connects us with the idea of consciousness that existed since the beginning, that has existed through all time, that is true, and that is the great enlightening teacher. This negates any negative energy that might be directed at you before it reaches your consciousness.

SHAME

What will give the healing is the flow of your soul energy.
YOGI BHAJAN

There is no room in the world for shame when love is present. Guilt and shame have nothing to do with spirituality. Shame is an inwardly toxifying emotion. It is one of most constricting feelings there is and one that the majority of human beings have experienced at one point or another. Shame is typically hidden away beneath a false persona, even a cheerful front, because shame actually masks the fear of nonacceptance. The ego likes to project a socially admirable facade. As that projection solidifies, we run the risk of losing the ability to access the authentic magnificence of our soul. We start to believe in the facade we have created.

Shame starts at an early age as we shrink back from being scolded, chastised, belittled, teased, bullied, ignored, or dismissed. We make ourselves small and become afraid of letting our effervescent selves be seen. Shame separates us from our higher selves and prevents us from allowing the gifts of the divine to flow with ease. Shame is a limiting belief that something is wrong with us, that we are not likeable enough or good enough to fit in with everyone else. Shame falsely tells us we are broken.

During this time on earth, we are evolving at such a rapid pace that we often find ourselves searching for a way to feel safe and grounded; we hunt for old, familiar forms of guidance. We are conflicted; we feel called to answer the direction of our hearts, yet we are confused by our feelings of shame. We hide our fear that we are not good enough. However, we must remember this truth: there is nothing wrong. We are all here on earth to evolve. We now find ourselves standing on our own two beautiful feet as agents of the divine. The wall between heaven and earth is no longer rigid. There are windows that let the breeze through, and when the wind of heaven touches our hearts, we are moved by grace. We feel our angelic nature as our reality and are in fact becoming angelic beings having very human experiences while at the same time questioning ourselves when we do not follow the rules of society. We often feel as if we are coloring outside of the lines and that there may be something wrong with us because we are not conforming to the life manual. This is the time to trust and have courage. Slowly but surely, the path of light and acceptance will open. Love will prevail over shame.

Shame is a toxin, and we are being called to detox from it. We are hearing the whispers of our ancestors asking us to please let the shame go and to step forward into the evolution of our lineage. Many of our ancestors felt shame, yet social restrictions were so severe that they did not have a safe outlet to release it. Shame was a private emotion. But it needs to be released, and at this time in our world we are recognizing together that when love is present, shame dissolves. We are being reminded to see beyond the illusion of false perfection.

Humanity is moving out of the age in which reason was held as an almost sacred motivation, leading to profit-making inventions, advances in pharmacology, heroes, stars, rulers, royalty, followers, fans, competition, and conditional love. We are entering a new paradigm—a time of service, love of all life, respect for self and others, cooperation, the experience of heaven on earth, sharing, caring, consciousness, gracefulness, heart-centered business, unconditional love, collective awareness, self-healing, and a new integrity through a developed consciousness. These are huge changes, and they are happening now. We sense the shift within ourselves as individuals and may feel isolated as a result. But many people are feeling the need to trust the divine as they experience it. The shame that has been ingrained in our subconscious minds is not something that can survive these transitions into our new world.

○ MEDITATION FOR RELEASING SHAME

When love is present, there is no duality. When love is present, we recognize that a force is moving through us. When love is present, we recognize that we are children of God who are cocreating a new world. This is a life without shame, a life full of passion, purpose, strength, grace, limitless potential, and surrender. This is the time for miracles.

The following meditation can help eliminate feelings of shame so that you can make space for the miracles that are seeking you. Do not do this exercise facing another person—face a landscape or visualize a vast horizon line instead. You can offer your meditation up to the earth, the sky, the wind, the air, the ocean, the mountains, the forest, or any naturally cleansing aspect of creation that you feel emotionally connected with.

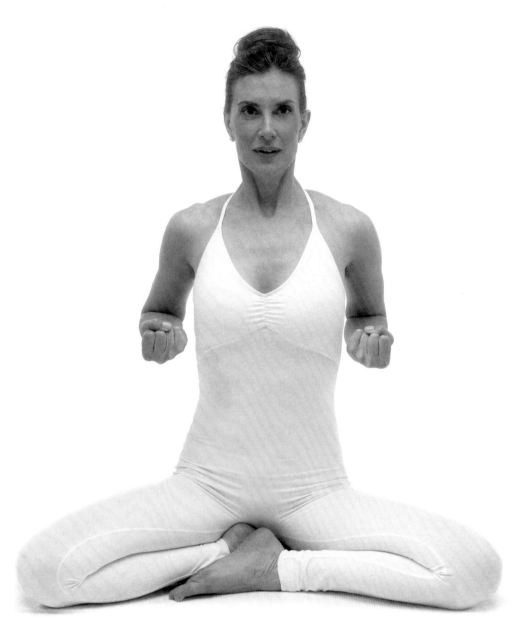

1 Sit in a cross-legged position and slow your breathing down, feeling the flow of air entering and exiting through your nostrils.

2 Make fists with your hands. Draw them back tightly toward your rib cage, so your elbows are bent and your upper arms are alongside your torso. Inhale deeply.

3 Exhale as you straighten one arm from the shoulder and twist the fist out in front of you. Focus your open eyes on one specific point, like a target that you are punching.

4 Inhale as you bend your elbow and draw the fist back to the shoulder.

5 Repeat the action with the other arm, using the same breath pattern.

6 Maintain the breathing pattern as you keep

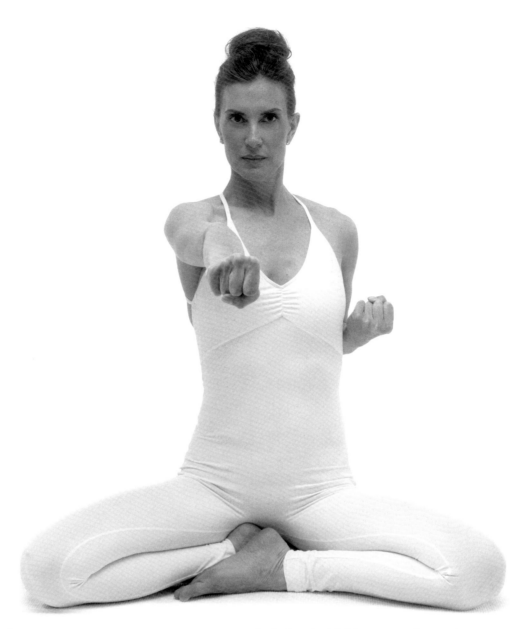

alternating arms, continuing at a rapid pace for one to five minutes. Move strongly from the shoulders. Shame is a combination of sadness and anger and often resides in the shoulders.

7 To finish, bring both fists back tightly alongside your rib cage, to the starting position, as you inhale deeply. Hold your breath and focus all your energy into your fists.

8 Exhale and raise both hands overhead. Shake your hands and arms vigorously as though you were shaking off dust. Breathe deeply as you shake for fifteen seconds, then release your arms down to rest on your knees. Transition back to normal breathing and feel a sense of gratitude for the release. Remember you are a soul made of pure light and pure love.

LISTENING TO THE STILL, SMALL VOICE WITHIN

The quieter you become, the more you can hear.
RAM DASS

The soul has a quiet voice. It is so quiet it often gets drowned out, yet it is so timeless it is content to wait. The ego and the mind, meanwhile, are shouting and impatient, full of bravado, coaxing us to jump to conclusions. As we contemplate our course of action, many times we are bombarded with thoughts. We strive for balance and for soul-level clarity, but competing voices argue inside our head, like a family loudly bickering in the apartment upstairs. Just like that loud family, the competing thoughts in our head can seem out of our control and keep us up at night. If we do sleep, we wake with our questions still unresolved.

Listening to the quiet voice of our soul requires two things: first, developing our delicately sensitive intuition while at the same strengthening our capacity to focus, and, second, holding that intuitive grace as a center point of our awareness. Intuition can be clearly developed with kundalini yoga practices. Once intuition is developed, we find the courage to act on it.

○ MEDITATION FOR GUIDANCE

There is a subtle line of energy that flows between our pineal and pituitary glands. It was known to the ancient yogis as the *golden cord*. That string of pure energy is so delicate that it vibrates with shifts in the electromagnetic field passing through it. Imagine the string of a violin that resonates more loudly or softly with emotion and feeling in accordance with the movement of a concert master's bow across it. In order for our intuition to function, it requires a stability and calm energy of both the pituitary and the pineal glands so as to energize and sensitize the golden cord.

The following meditation enhances the subtle radiance between our pineal and pituitary glands, activating our intuition. It brings an inner silence from which deep, soul-motivated action can spring forth. A peace comes over our thoughts, and in the freedom we can discern the clear, quiet, honest voice of our timeless soul.

This meditation has two phases: first a breathing exercise (in which the mantra is chanted silently) and then a period of chanting out loud. The mantra "Waho Guru" (pronounced "*wah*-hoh guh-*roo*") opens us to the wonder and acceptance of this divine guidance.

In the first phase, the use of the Segmented Breath technique (described in detail in chapter 4) activates the pituitary gland. The bowl-shaped mudra you make at the heart center opens our psyche to receive guidance our soul. We invite you to visualize your body as a sacred place that receives the blessings of the divine. You may want to have a notebook by your side, so you can write down the messages you hear right after the chanting phase.

Waho Guru

1 Sit up with a straight spine on the floor or in a chair. Observe the flow of your breathing through your nostrils and notice the expansion and contraction of your rib cage with each breath. Feel the exquisite sensation of your spine rising up from the pelvis to the top of your head.

2 Bend your elbows and form a bowl with your hands in front of your heart, holding the sides of the pinkies slightly apart to create a fish-shaped gap between them.

3 Tip your head slightly forward toward the bowl, almost as though it might fall in, elongating your neck.

4 Lower your eyelids down until they are almost closed and gaze into the bowl you have made. We invite you to look into the radiance of your hands and imagine that you will be receiving a gift, the gift of prasad, the blessing of the infinite.

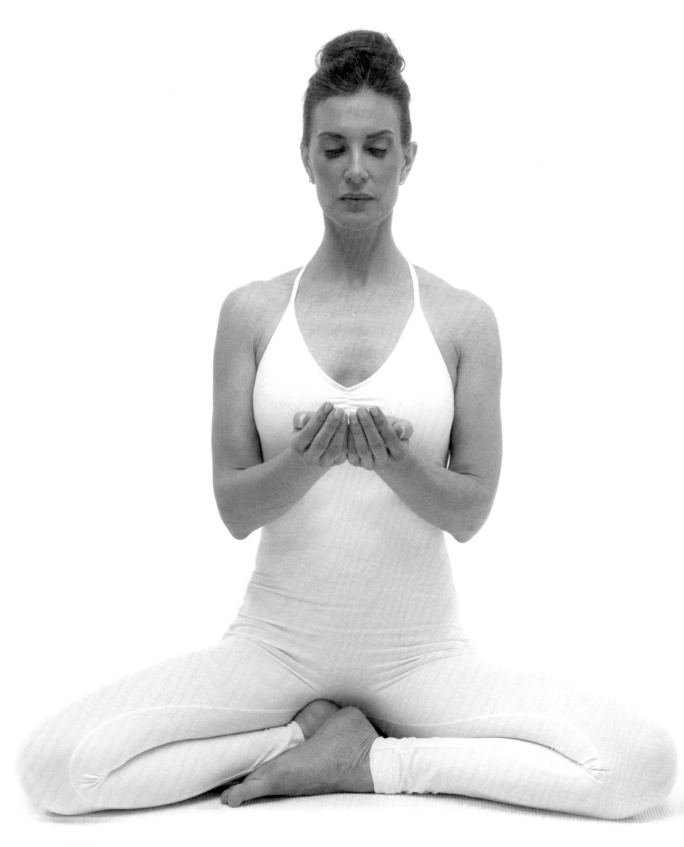

5 Inhale through your nose, dividing your breath into ten sniffs of equal length (not eight, as in the original instruction in chapter 4) to form the Segmented Breath. Rather than constricting the throat, create each little sniff with an internal tug on the diaphragm. Find the right volume of air so that by the tenth sniff your lungs are totally full and your rib cage is expanded. On each of the ten sniffs, mentally vibrate the first sound of the mantra, "wah-hoh," as if you were hearing it silently in your mind.

6 When you are ready to empty your lungs, divide the exhalation into ten equal parts, each done with a little movement of the diaphragm. Find the right volume of air for each so that your lungs are fully emptied by the tenth exhalation. On each of the ten exhalations, mentally vibrate the second sound of the mantra, "Guru."

7 Continue this combination of breathing, mantra, and visualization for three to eleven minutes.

8 Inhale deeply to finish this first portion of the meditation, then exhale with a single powerful breath, expelling all the air from your lungs. Transition without pause to the next portion of the meditation.

9 Keep the same posture— sitting up straight, hands making the bowl shape, head reaching toward the bowl, and eyelids lowered—but now begin to chant the mantra aloud. Chant the first word eight times: "Waho, Waho, Waho, Waho, Waho, Waho, Waho, Waho." Then chant the second word eight times: "Guru, Guru, Guru, Guru, Guru, Guru, Guru, Guru." Chant at your own pace, steadily and in a monotone. Let your breath be natural, letting it come and go as needed.

Waho Guru

10 Keep the rhythm going steadily, chanting out loud for three to thirty-one minutes, or longer if you like, vibrating the sound through your spine and through your aura.

11 To finish, inhale deeply and suspend your breath. Then exhale fully and hold out the breath. Relax your hands onto your knees as you transition to normal breathing, staying in a state of openness and receptivity. Don't rush off. This is the moment you have been waiting for. Now ask the infinite that moves through you for clarity; ask for guidance from your soul. Take your time and allow the divine to flow through you without judgment.

12 Once you feel the guidance is complete, thank the divine. Recognize it as coming from you. Thank your soul.

HIGH-FREQUENCY SLEEP

Deep sleep is a powerful opportunity for cleansing our mind of thoughts that do not serve us. However, today's world is moving at such an accelerated pace that even after eight hours we have not always reached the deepest levels of restoration that we need in order to feel healthy and refreshed. If we drift off to sleep thinking of the difficulties of the day and worrying about the challenges ahead, we trigger the release of stress hormones and suppress the calming action of the parasympathetic nervous system, short-circuiting a powerful opportunity for restoring the perfect health and alignment of our mind, body, and spirit. Our energetic vibration just before falling asleep keeps circulating throughout our aura all through the night. It is the thoughts we think just before dropping off that we marinate in all night long, intensifying as we sleep.

Many people are having a hard time falling asleep and staying asleep these days because our nervous systems are in overdrive. With all the medical advancements we have made in the last hundred years, it is quite bewildering to see how many people are struggling with relaxation. Is the problem too much technology? Is it the stress of the collective consciousness? Whatever it is, our job is to "be the change we wish to see in the world," as the saying goes. Start with your own healing and let it become a lighthouse for others.

During your prebedtime routine and before closing your eyes, remember that you are grace, you are love, you are worthy of all good things, and you are much more loved than you can even imagine. Repeat these internal messages from your soul to yourself. These affirmations will increase your vibratory frequency and help you sleep.

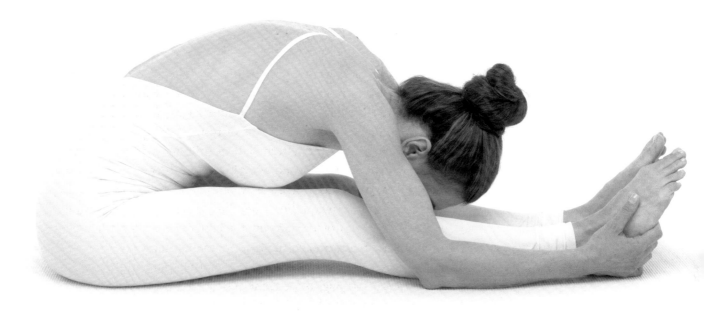

○ THE ELIXIR FOR CALM

Breathing through the left nostril is a beautiful way to bring yourself to a state of peace. When we rest in a pose of surrender before practicing left nostril breathing, our entire being relaxes. Seated Forward Bends gently stimulate the parasympathetic nervous system, calming the stress response, and are a great tool for quieting the mind. We developed this sequence for people who have a hard time unwinding and getting to sleep after a stressful day.

1　Sit on the ground with your legs extended out in front of you. Fold your torso over your legs in a Seated Forward Bend. Breathe deeply. Let all the tension dissolve from your shoulders as if a waterfall is releasing everything that is bothering you. Hold this pose for at least one full minute.

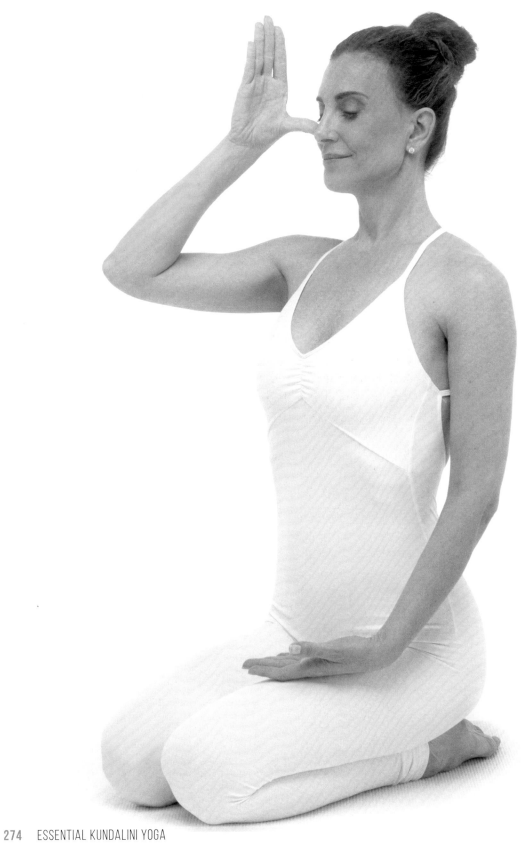

2 Now sit up in a comfortable position, either cross-legged on the floor, on a chair, or in your bed. Bring your right thumb to your right nostril and direct all the other fingers of your right hand up toward the sky. Our fingers are like antennas connecting us to the angelic realm.

3 Inhale through your left nostril for a count of four.

4 Hold your breath for a count of four.

5 Exhale slowly for a count of four.

6 Hold the breath out for a count of four.

7 Continue this breathing pattern for three minutes. Begin to feel how this cooling breath calms your nervous system. Trust that angels are rubbing your back and whispering peaceful sounds to you. Trust that you are safe and all is well. Trust that there is an order to this universe even in times of chaos.

8 Lie down in your bed. Imagine yourself in a very comforting place with angels to your left, angels to your right, angels above you, and angels below you. Be still and know you have a thousand angels with you. Shhhhhhh. Sleep. All is well.

ACTIVATING HEALING

When the prayer becomes the vibration of the soul,
mind, and self we can create a miracle.
YOGI BHAJAN

Attention is a concentrated direction of energy. Healing is an optimization of genetic expression for our highest good. Our power is our connection with grace. And sound vibrates intention into matter. When we put these four principles together, we become a powerhouse for bringing about healing. Distance makes no difference because in the quantum world, when a vibration occurs in one place, it will vibrate simultaneously with any harmonically resonant particle in another place. When we clear the aura and then allow our prayer to vibrate in our aura, it will resonate powerfully and continue into the infinite.

○ MEDITATION FOR HEALING SELF AND OTHERS

Ra
Ma
Da
Sa
Sa Say
So
Hung

The ancient mantra "Ra Ma Da Sa Sa Say So Hung" (pronounced "raa maa daa saa saa say so hung") consists of eight syllables that vibrate the atoms of the physical world with the resonance of healing. These sounds work in conjunction with nature. They stimulate our DNA to express its most healing qualities. The principle is to focus our awareness on the most delicate and subtle vibrations in and around us and to make the choice to vibrate love with the grace of the universe flowing through us. You can chant this mantra for three minutes, eleven minutes, or thirty-one minutes—the traditional sacred amounts of time—or for any length of time at all. Even when things seem hopeless, try this mantra. Our translation of the mantra is:

Ra "sun"

Ma "moon"

Da "earth"

Sa "merger of earth into infinity"

Sa Say "creative totality"

So "merger of body and soul"

Hung "vibrating into the heavens"

The following meditation combines the healing power of this mantra with a sacred meditative movement to generate a deeply powerful force for healing ourselves and others.

1   Sit up straight, close your eyes, and focus internally on the third eye point. Feel your breath flowing in and out through your nose, stimulating and bringing prana deeply into your body. Bring all your attention to feeling the joy of the healing as though you had just gotten a phone call telling you that all is well. Tangibly experience what that feels like to you and stay with it.

2   Bring your hands out in front of you with palms up and your elbows bent slightly so your forearms are parallel to the ground and a little angled to the sides. Imagine you are ready for an embrace. Please see photo on the following page.

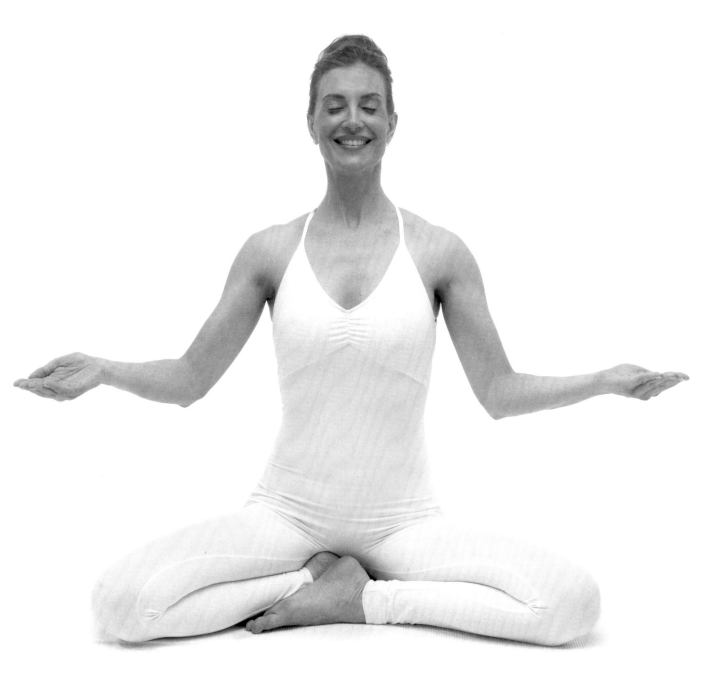

3 Slowly and gracefully bring the hands toward your chest, as though you are scooping up energy, stopping at a point about six inches in front of your heart.

4 Return to the original position as described in step 2 and continue slowly and gracefully scooping the energy of nature toward your heart and rib cage. The movement is soft and gentle.

5 Begin to chant the mantra "Ra Ma Da Sa Sa Sey So Hung" out loud. Allow each syllable to arise freely and vibrate your skull and spinal cord. On the final syllable, "Hung," pull

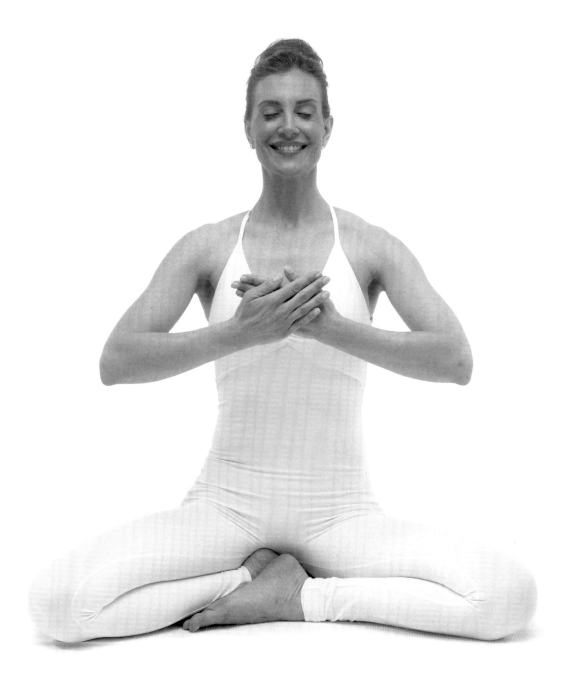

the navel inward and powerfully vibrate the upper palate, midbrain, and top of the skull with the sound. It should feel buzzy.

6 To finish, bring your hands to your knees. Inhale deeply and focus all your intention. Then exhale and relax your breath. Stay with the energy for as long as you can before you rise and continue with your day. Feel the healing force of nature coursing through your cells. Pray for those you need and give them access to this infinite flowing energy. Allow, trust, and believe.

GETTING OLDER

As the decades go by, we enter into a wise, beautiful time—the time to tap into elevation and expansion. Our DNA holds the ability to rebuild our cells for our entire lives, but scientists do not yet understand why we seem to lose the capacity to rebuild, renew, and repair our body with age. The market for hormones, antioxidants, age-defying lotions, and plastic surgery is massive, yet none of these fixes has been able to help anyone hold on to the actual vitality of youth. In the process of staying alive, our body slowly but surely accumulates the toxic by-products of our very own cellular metabolism, and these then appear to take a toll on our cellular regeneration. It's as though we don't take out the trash on a regular basis, and after a while, it starts to fill up the kitchen.

It's interesting to note, however, that the ancient yogis often lived for a very long time, staying healthy and vigorous until their last breaths. This is because kundalini yoga focuses on charging the magnetic environment of our DNA, hormone optimization, and the removal of toxins—physical, mental, emotional, and spiritual—from our body and our energy field. As we've discussed, the electromagnetic field that our DNA operates within has a dramatic effect on how our genes are expressed. And the hormonal balance that kundalini yoga generates in the pituitary and pineal glands optimizes the state of all the glands in the body. The core principles are regular yoga practice, Deep Relaxation, and the Love Frequency Phenomenon for health. Remember, when our prana vibrates at a frequency of love, our entire being, from the physical body to our emotions, operates at its highest potential.

○ THE LONGEVITY KRIYA

A few kriyas are so powerful and are said to work so effectively that they should be practiced for only nine minutes at a time to achieve a powerful effect. The Longevity Kriya is one of them. This kriya uses three unique hand positions to generate subtle shifts in your electromagnetic field and to stimulate energy channels that run through the shoulders and elbows. Start with one minute for each position and build up to a maximum of three minutes each.

If the Longevity Kriya is practiced nine minutes a day for forty days, it is said that the molecular structure of the physical body can heal. It keeps the DNA intact and directly stimulates the vagus nerve and the brain stem for hormonal balance. It can help you release and transform addictive thoughts and distress and can effectively alter your mind-set from negative to positive. The results can be quite dramatic.

○ 1 TUNING IN

Sit up with your spine straight. Feel the flow of breath bringing energy into your body. Chant the Adi Mantra.

Ong
Namo
Guru
Dev
Namo

○ 2 INDEX FINGER MUDRA

1 Raise your right arm up to sixty degrees in front of you. Point your left arm downward behind you in a sixty-degree angle. Imagine you are forming a straight sixty-degree line with your arms, like an arrow.

2 Turn your right palm down and your left palm up. Make a pointing mudra with both hands, extending the index finger and folding your other fingers into your palm, crossing your thumbs over your middle finger. Point the index fingers and the arrow in opposite directions and push your index fingers apart to elongate your arms from the shoulders, making the distance between your fingertips as long as possible. Keep your elbows locked straight, feeling a straight line of energy running between the fingertips of your right and left hands.

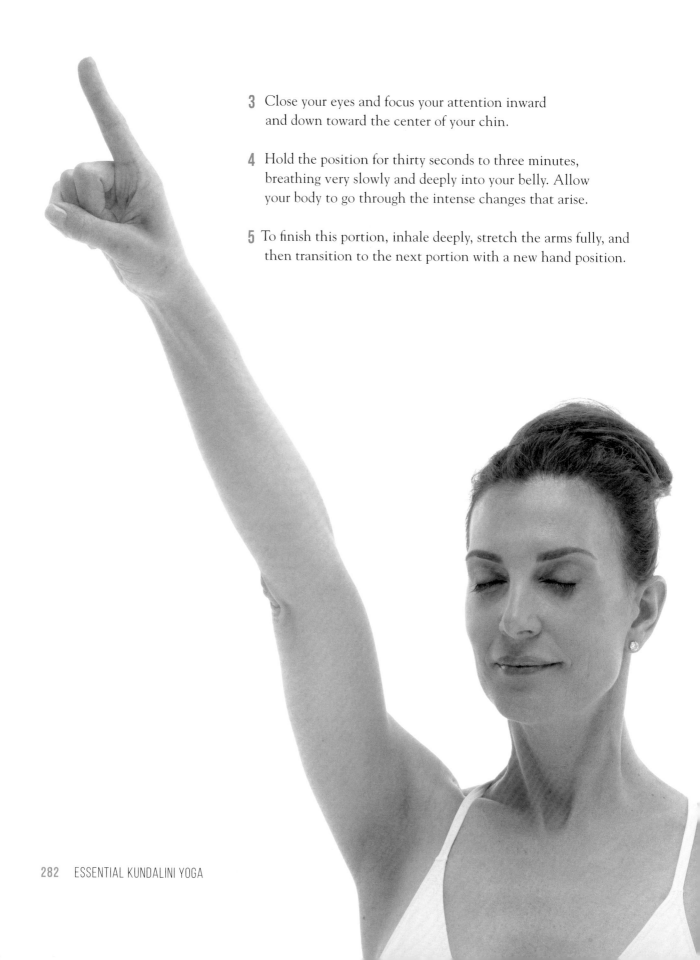

3 Close your eyes and focus your attention inward and down toward the center of your chin.

4 Hold the position for thirty seconds to three minutes, breathing very slowly and deeply into your belly. Allow your body to go through the intense changes that arise.

5 To finish this portion, inhale deeply, stretch the arms fully, and then transition to the next portion with a new hand position.

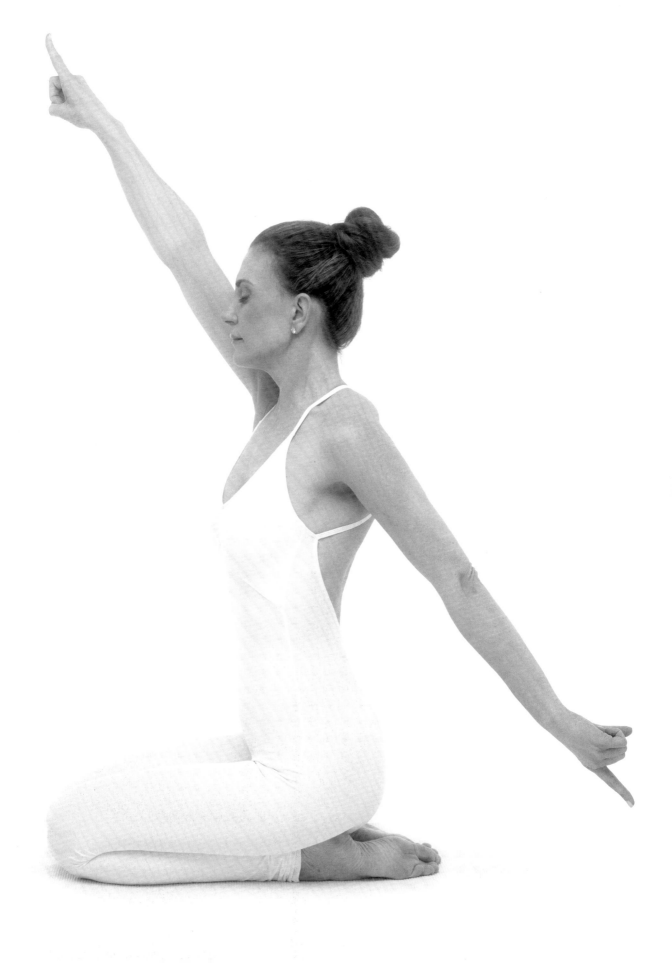

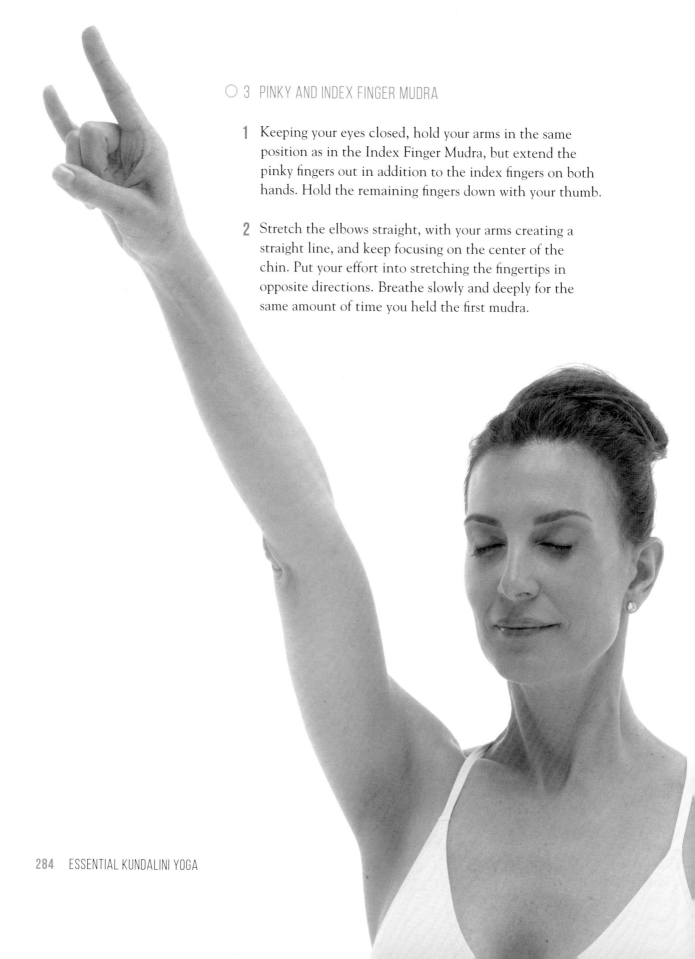

○ 3 PINKY AND INDEX FINGER MUDRA

1 Keeping your eyes closed, hold your arms in the same position as in the Index Finger Mudra, but extend the pinky fingers out in addition to the index fingers on both hands. Hold the remaining fingers down with your thumb.

2 Stretch the elbows straight, with your arms creating a straight line, and keep focusing on the center of the chin. Put your effort into stretching the fingertips in opposite directions. Breathe slowly and deeply for the same amount of time you held the first mudra.

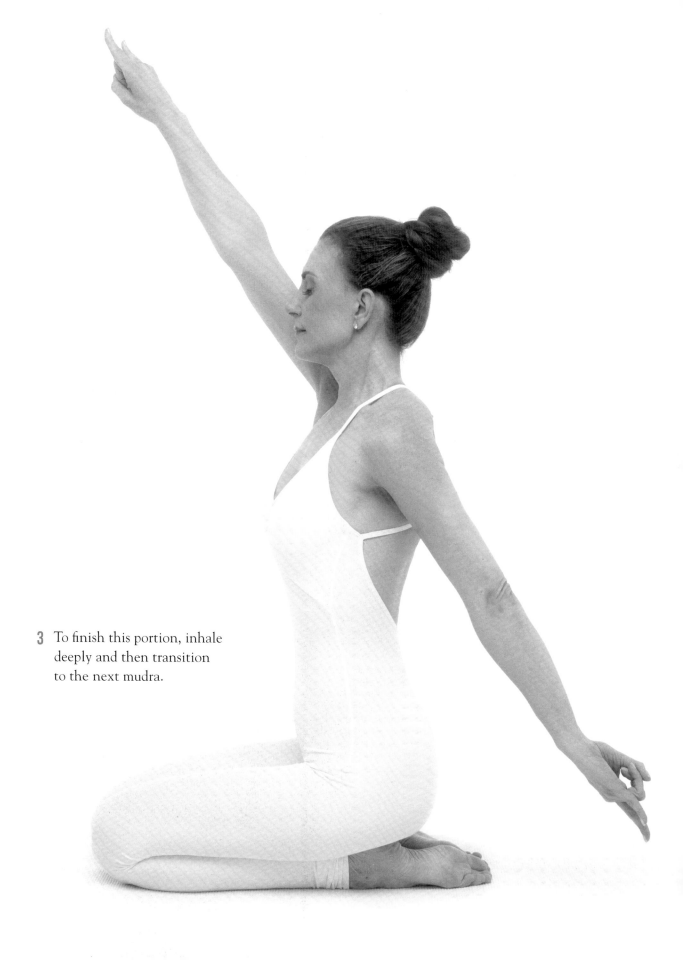

3 To finish this portion, inhale
deeply and then transition
to the next mudra.

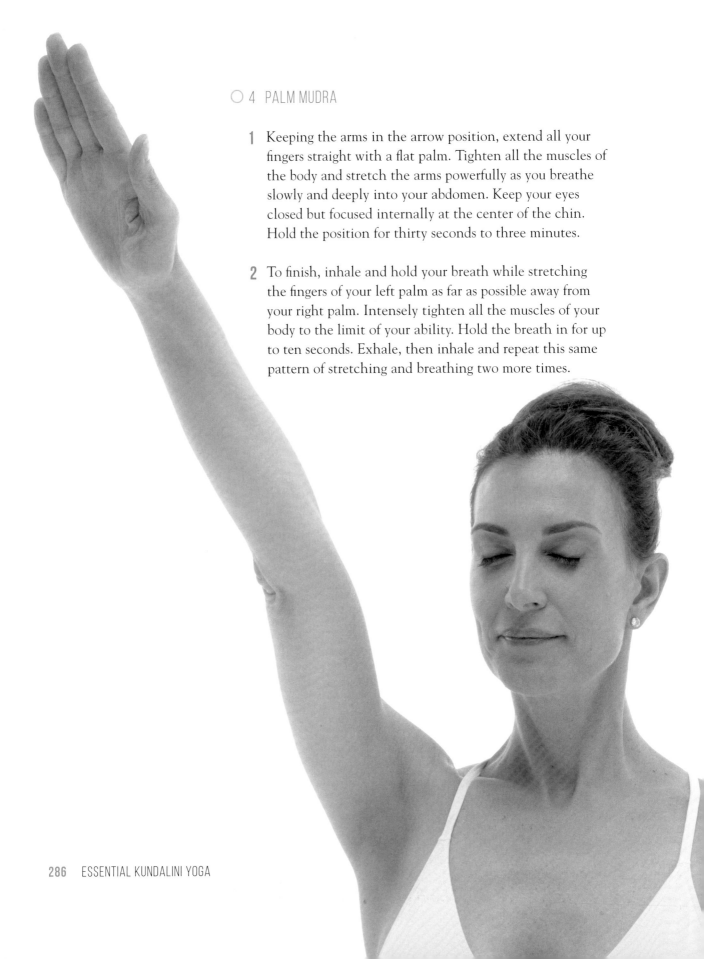

○ 4 PALM MUDRA

1   Keeping the arms in the arrow position, extend all your
    fingers straight with a flat palm. Tighten all the muscles of
    the body and stretch the arms powerfully as you breathe
    slowly and deeply into your abdomen. Keep your eyes
    closed but focused internally at the center of the chin.
    Hold the position for thirty seconds to three minutes.

2   To finish, inhale and hold your breath while stretching
    the fingers of your left palm as far as possible away from
    your right palm. Intensely tighten all the muscles of your
    body to the limit of your ability. Hold the breath in for up
    to ten seconds. Exhale, then inhale and repeat this same
    pattern of stretching and breathing two more times.

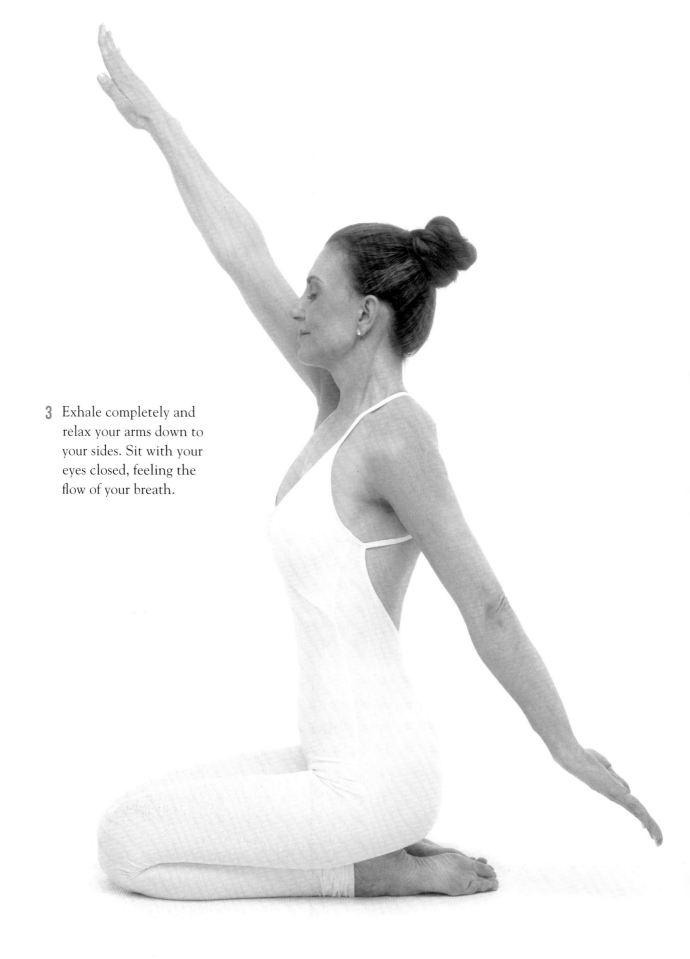

3 Exhale completely and relax your arms down to your sides. Sit with your eyes closed, feeling the flow of your breath.

Rest on your back. Feel the energy of rejuvenation and joy flowing into every cell in your body, awakening your genes to heal, restore, and express your highest potential.

SHAKING OFF SADNESS

Sometimes in life we feel sad without even knowing why. We feel the weight of sadness as a heaviness on the skin that we are unable to shake off. Sadness can be caused by a misalignment or a tear in our electromagnetic field. When our energy field is weak, we can feel influenced by other energies that may not support our greater good. This can happen to those who are deeply connected with higher dimensions. One simple solution is to purify our energy field by chanting the Mul Mantra out loud. You can find about the Mul Mantra in chapter 5. Another is the powerful meditation below.

○ COLD DEPRESSION MEDITATION

Sometimes life is complicated. We may be able to cope with everyday stresses, but when we have multiple traumatic events happening at once, we can feel frozen by fear and uncertainty, stuck in our painful circumstances. We may feel victimized and incapable of making a move. As our modern age speeds up, this feeling can intensify to the point that we make ourselves sick. What can we do when we feel so confused and empty that we become immobilized and exhausted?

This kundalini meditation is designed to help center your consciousness and channel all your confusion out of your psyche. You give your feelings of uncertainty, pain, and blame to the universe and replace them with the pure, clear light of your soul, accessing what was actually there all along.

Ek Ong Kar

Sat Nam

Kartaa Purkh

Nirbhao

Nirvair

Akaal Moorat

Ajoonee

Saibhang

Gur Prasaad

Jap

Aad Sach

Jugaad Sach

Hai Bhee Sach

Nanak Hosee Bhee

Sach

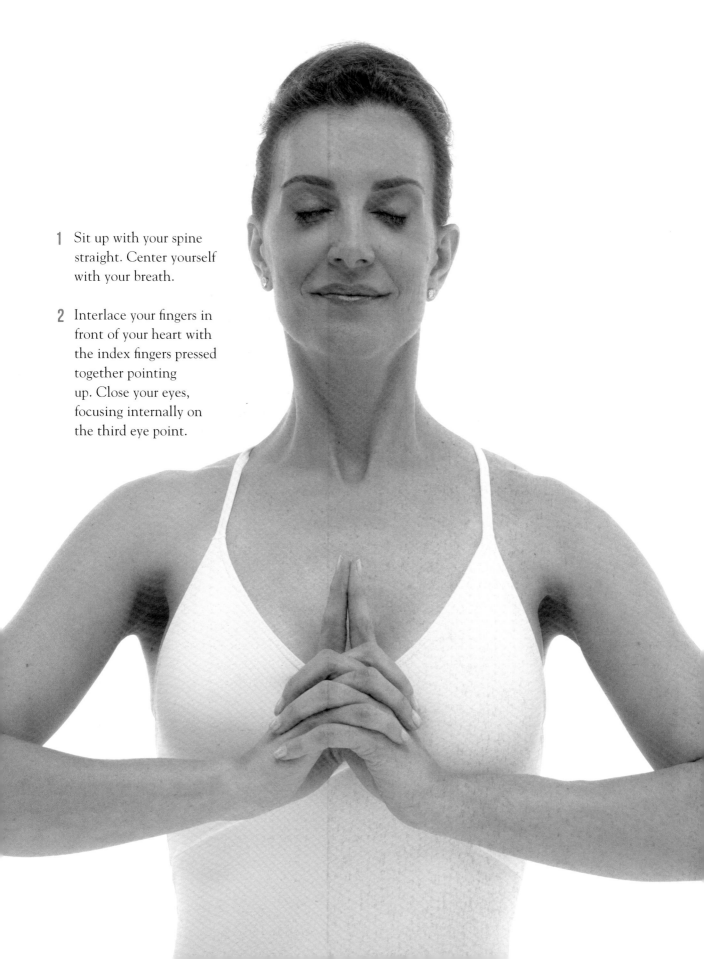

1 Sit up with your spine
straight. Center yourself
with your breath.

2 Interlace your fingers in
front of your heart with
the index fingers pressed
together pointing
up. Close your eyes,
focusing internally on
the third eye point.

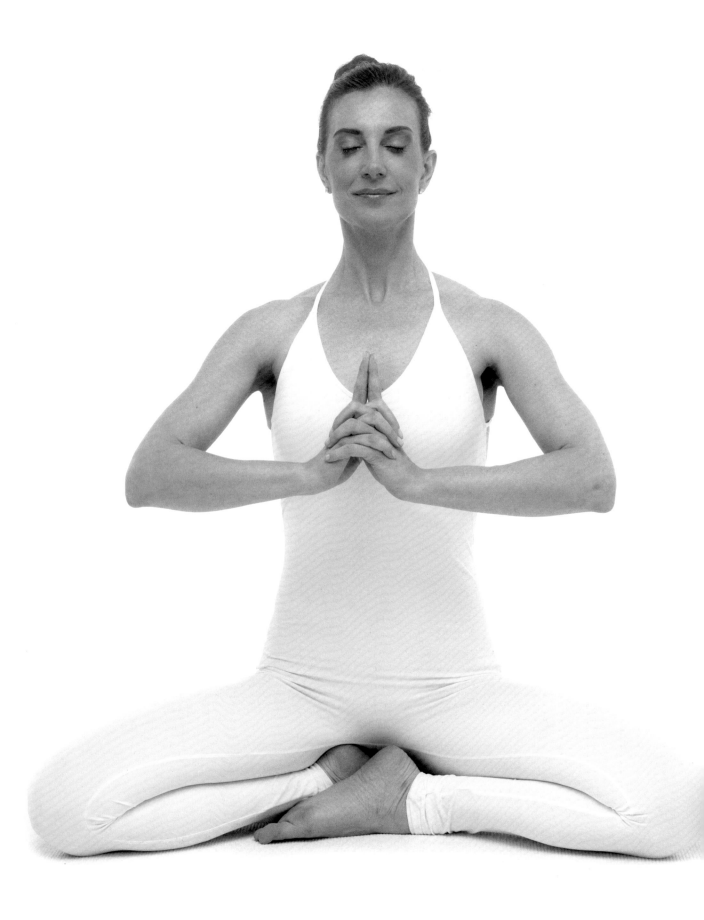

3 Begin chanting the mantra "Wahe Guru, Wahe Guru, Wahe Guru, Wahe Jio" (pronounced "*wah*-hey guh-roo, *wah*-hey guh-roo, *wah*-hey guh-roo, *wah*-hey jee-oh"). Our translation of this mantra is: "As in amazement, here and now, all darkness is transformed to illuminating light in my soul." Practice doing this chant with the following visualization:

Wahe Guru
Wahe Guru
Wahe Guru
Wahe Jio

- On the syllable of "wah," feel the sound vibrating at your navel.

- On the syllable of "hey," feel the sound vibrating at your heart.

- On the syllables of "gur-roo" and "jee-oh," feel the sounds vibrating at your lips.

4 Continue chanting the mantra for up to eleven minutes.

5 Inhale deeply and hold your breath in. Feel the echo of the sounds still vibrating in your navel, heart, and lips. Suspend your breath for as long as you comfortably can and then exhale very consciously.

6 Inhale a second time and again suspend your breath. Release the feeling of being trapped by circumstances. Surrender it to the universe. Surrender your pain and feelings of blame. Release your stress and your uncertainty. Give it all to God. Hold the breath for as long as you comfortably can and then exhale, still holding your concentration.

7 Inhale a third time and give your life to God. Surrender. Whatever God means to you, offer your existence to that. Allow yourself to feel the purification this action creates in your psyche. When you are ready, exhale and sit for a while with the whole experience of this powerful meditation.

COURAGE TO SHINE

If we honestly ask ourselves what in our day-to-day life prevents us from expressing the pure love at the core of our being, the answer is always fear. We hide our true selves to fit in, to be polite, and to avoid offending anyone. Rather than encouraging ourselves to transform, we find comfort in conforming to a world that is struggling. To break free of our challenges, we must be willing to live in our authentic expression of truth. This is our "Sat Nam," the genuine truth of our manifestation vibrating at its highest frequency.

We are a new creation. All of us. It may be beyond our state of comprehension to acknowledge this in our minds, but our hearts know this truth. We are glowing and growing as a species, and it is essential that we do not fall back into entrenched patterns of fear. The inner light we tap into in quiet moments of connection to the soul is a reminder of the love the universe feels for us. Sometimes all we need is a few minutes to bring ourselves back into the quiet connection.

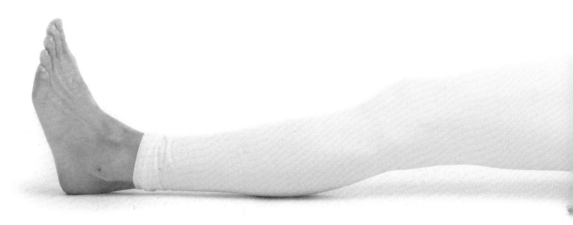

○ KUNDALINI YOGA TO DISSOLVE THE BARRIERS OF FEAR

Most of the things we fear are not real. Most of the things we fear never in fact happen. Fear is an emotion that gets stuck in the mind and resonates in our aura. It stimulates our sympathetic nervous system to go on high alert, and this takes a long time to settle back out of. The response to fear is hardwired into us from our cave person evolution, but the calling of the modern age is how to be courageous in living our truth as spiritual beings while we still carry the genes for survival from tiger attacks in every cell of our body.

The following set is a quick and potent one that works on releasing accumulated effects of fear that constrict the flow of energy through the life nerve, vagus nerve, and aura. It helps shake off the energetic debris that holds us back from living to our highest, fullest potential.

1 Lie on your back. Lift your left leg up in the air and shake it vigorously for one to three minutes. Lower it down. Lift the right leg up and shake it vigorously for the same length of time.

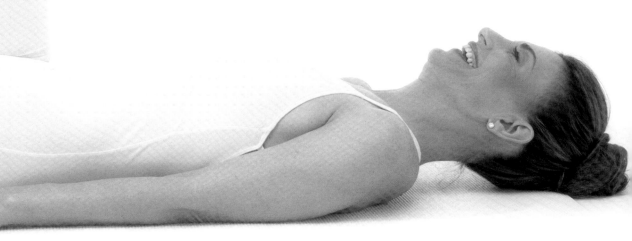

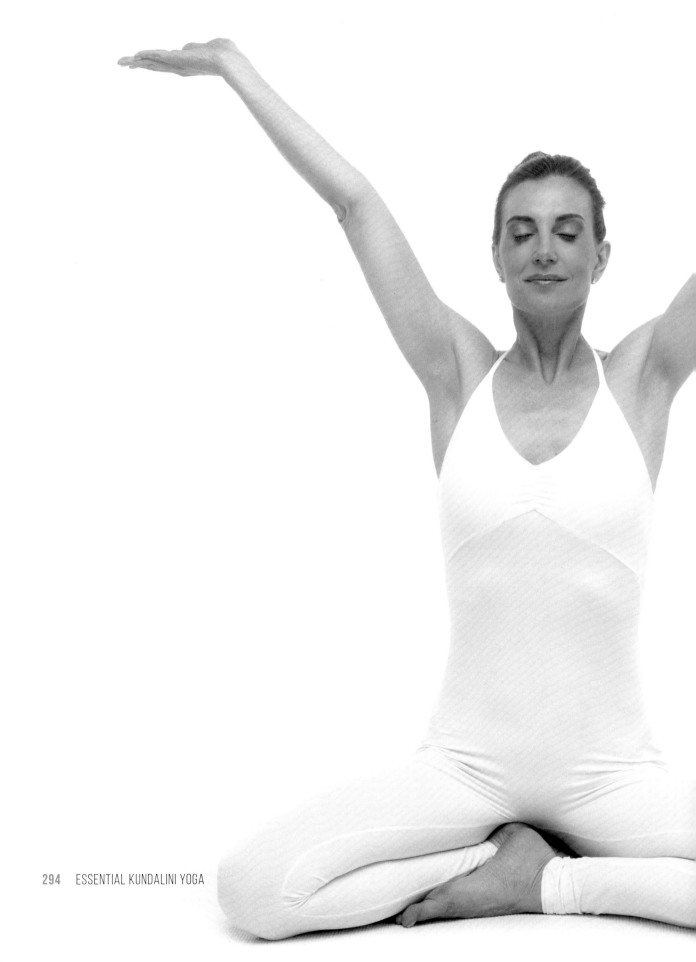

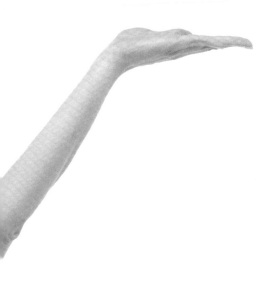

2 Come up to a seated position. Reach your arms up to sixty
   degrees on either side of your head, creating a V shape. Open
   your palms toward the sky and flop the hands open from the
   wrists. Breathe deeply and gaze at the tip of your nose. Feel
   yourself receiving the light of the divine while you surrender
   any barriers you hold inside. Let go. Continue for three minutes.

3 Bring your arms down, breathe gently, and relax. Feel yourself
   opening and allowing the full magnificence of your soul to shine.

YOGA FOR FERTILITY

Conceiving a child is a miracle. Sometimes it can take time and nurturing for pregnancy to occur. Kundalini yoga is a wonderful tool for conscious conception for both men and women. It integrates the spiritual, energetic, conscious, and unconscious aspects of a person as well as strengthening the nervous system, balancing the hormonal system, and energizing the muscles, organs, and joints of the physical body.

While all of the chakras come into play, it is essential to have a balanced second chakra in order for healthy conception to happen. Many men and women feel as though they are running on adrenaline, weakening their sexuality, sensuality, sensitivity, and emotional well-being. They lose touch with the natural balance that comes from aligning with the creative embrace of the universe.

○ **MIRACLE MANTRA FOR FERTILITY**

Oncologists and reproductive endocrinologists are using sound healing modalities as an adjunct to Western medicine with excellent results. Sacred sound adds another dimension that can truly alter your brain chemistry, hormonal balance, and nervous system.

*Guru Guru
Wahe Guru
Guru Guru
Ram Das Guru*

1 To support your fertility, chant the Miracle Mantra "Guru Guru Wahe Guru, Guru Guru Ram Das Guru" (described in chapter 5) for three to eleven minutes every day upon waking. Do not worry about how to chant the mantra. Simply allow the sound and the words to flow from you freely.

2 When you finish chanting, sit in focused gratitude. Remember that gratitude lifts your energetic vibration so you can attract your dreams. If you feel stuck, begin with small thoughts of gratitude and allow the momentum to build.

○ FOUR EXERCISES FOR FERTILITY

Here are four exercises we've developed that help rebalance the second chakra so that creative expression and our natural, robust fertility are aligned with the ripe possibility of conception. These exercises work for both men and women, helping them to open, allow, and drop their resistance to the natural creativity of the universe flowing through them.

○ LONG, DEEP BREATHING

1 Sit up comfortably with your spine straight. As you inhale through your nose, visualize your breath as a white light coming down your spine, expanding your belly.

2 On the exhale, visualize your breath as light coming up the front of your body and out the nose. Gently deflate the belly as you exhale.

3 Continue this practice of white-light activation in conjunction with the breath for three minutes.

4 Now begin to visualize your belly as an orange balloon and let the balloon expand as you inhale and deflate as you exhale. Continue for one minute or longer. If you can sit with this visualization and breathing exercise for eleven minutes every single morning, you will notice a transformation in your creativity on many levels.

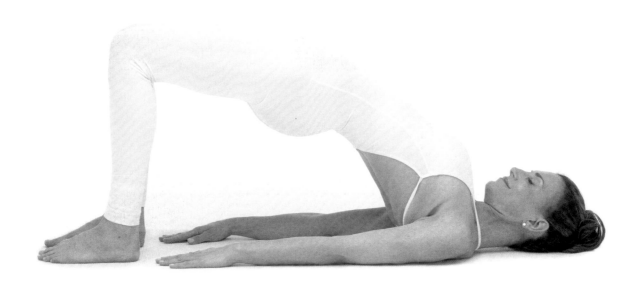

○ PELVIC LIFTS

1 Lie down on your back with your knees bent and your feet flat on the floor, the heels close to your buttocks. Press the bottoms of your feet and the palms of your hands into the floor. At the same time feel your belly softening and flowing with the breath, like a boat floating along the ocean.

2 Inhale as you raise your hips and buttocks up toward the sky and exhale as you lower them down to the starting position. Practice this breath-led movement for thirty seconds to three minutes.

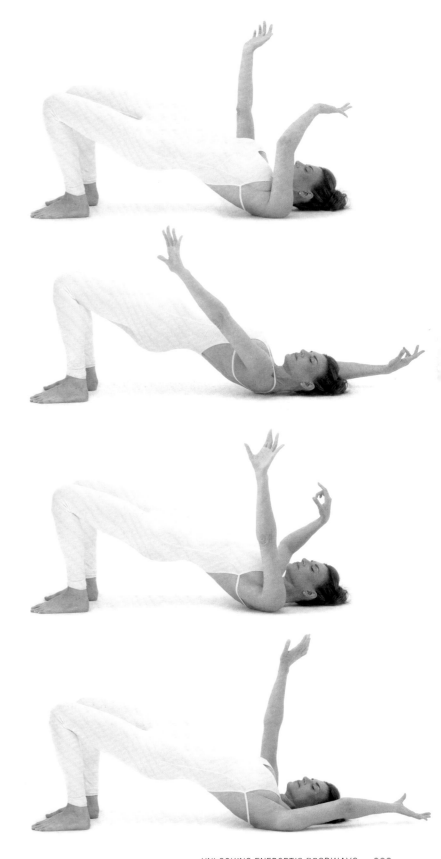

○ FERTILITY DANCE

1 In the same position, raise
   the hips up while arching
   your back; inhale and exhale
   deeply. Start dancing your
   hips, belly, and arms in
   the air. Lift your arms and
   incorporate them into the
   dance, allowing them to
   move freely. Be one with
   the flow of your breath.
   Let go of everything the
   mind tells you and release
   yourself into the movement.

2 Continue this movement
   for as long as you
   feel comfortable.

3 To finish, inhale deeply and
   lift your pelvis up as high
   as possible while holding
   your breath. Exhale and
   lower your spine to the
   ground one vertebra at a
   time. Rest on your back
   and let go of striving. Stop
   doing and simply be.

Lie on your back and visualize your healthy body attracting your spirit baby. Send love out from your heart and express your readiness for your baby to arrive. Connect with the energy field flowing in and around the space of your body. Know that you are healthy and affirm it by saying aloud, "My body is healthy, ready, and able to conceive."

BUNS OF LIGHT

The physical exercises in this book will certainly tone your body and help you shed extra pounds. There is nothing greater for toning the body than opening the energetic pathways while engaging various muscle groups. However, the physical exercises in yoga are but a small component of the full practice. If you think of a tree and all its branches, the physical postures would be one of the branches on the tree. *Yoga* means "to yoke body, mind, breath, and soul." We have worked out in gyms with weights; we have hiked, biked, and exercised in various other ways. While all exercise is great, there is a magnetic resonance that happens when we integrate the breath and the energy body with the physical body through kundalini yoga.

The yogic way to tone the glutes is by engaging the muscles in the backs of your thighs and buttocks while breathing deeply, allowing the breath to open any pranic blocks, and applying Root Lock to energize from the pelvic floor. We often carry a great deal of tension in our glutes, which translates into stagnant energy.

When that tension releases and prana can move freely again, your muscles develop a relaxed and strong tone that energetically expresses attractive, glowing health.

It is a misconception that we need to practice heavy exercise to maintain a healthy weight and lifestyle. Weight lifting will have a lesser effect if the glandular system is not in balance and if the sympathetic nervous system is in a perpetual state of alert. We have to relax and move in a way that allows our energy to course with joy and sensitivity. If we are eating healthy foods and getting enough exercise while keeping our cortisol levels balanced, the body will naturally maintain a healthy weight. Our metabolism shifts dramatically when we balance our glandular system, nervous system, and mind-body connection through yoga and meditation. Exercise alone does not have the magical impact that toning the physical body combined with breath, movement, and flowing energy provides. When we combine deep yogic breathing, the release of blocked energy in the first and second chakras, and rhythmic movement of the physical body, the effect is fantastic. Freeing the prana opens the flow of oxygen to the cells and helps eliminate cellulite. When we utilize meditative movement with a sense of relaxation in the midst of what can be an intense physical workout, astonishing transformation happens—and our bodies glow from top to bottom.

This book has a number of wonderful kundalini yoga exercises that will help tone your glutes and allow the prana of the first and second chakras to move. Pelvic Lifts (chapter 2 and this chapter), Frog Pose (chapter 7), and the Fertility Dance (this chapter) are all especially good for these purposes. Here are some of our other favorites.

○ TRIANGLE POSE WITH REVERSE LEG LIFTS

There are those days when we are traveling or busy working, commuting, parenting, and otherwise keeping up with the demands of life. This exercise can be practiced in a few minutes on the days when we simply do not have time for a full yoga practice, an hour at the gym, or a walk outside. This is a great exercise to do after you've been sitting for a while as well. Taking three minutes out of your day to practice this pose is more beneficial than you can imagine. It integrates mind, body, energy, and breath with the present moment.

1 Come onto your hands and knees on the floor, with your knees directly under your hips and your wrists directly below your shoulders. Press your hands into the floor, curl your toes under, and lift your buttocks up into Downward Facing Dog, with your weight balanced between your hands and feet.

2 As you inhale, lift your right heel up high behind you, pointing your toes.

3 As you exhale, bring the toes down to touch the ground.

4 Maintaining Downward Facing Dog, continue lifting your legs alternately for a total of twenty-six lifts. End with your left leg up in the air.

5 Keep your leg up, inhale, and begin Breath of Fire. Visualize a line of energy flowing unimpeded from your hands on the ground to your toes in the air as you do Breath of Fire for thirty seconds to three minutes.

6 Inhale deeply, hold the position as your energy dissolves through any blocks, and then lower your leg as you exhale.

7 Repeat steps 5 and 6 with the right leg held up.

8 To finish, lower yourself down and relax on your back. Breathe and feel the fresh flow of prana through your body.

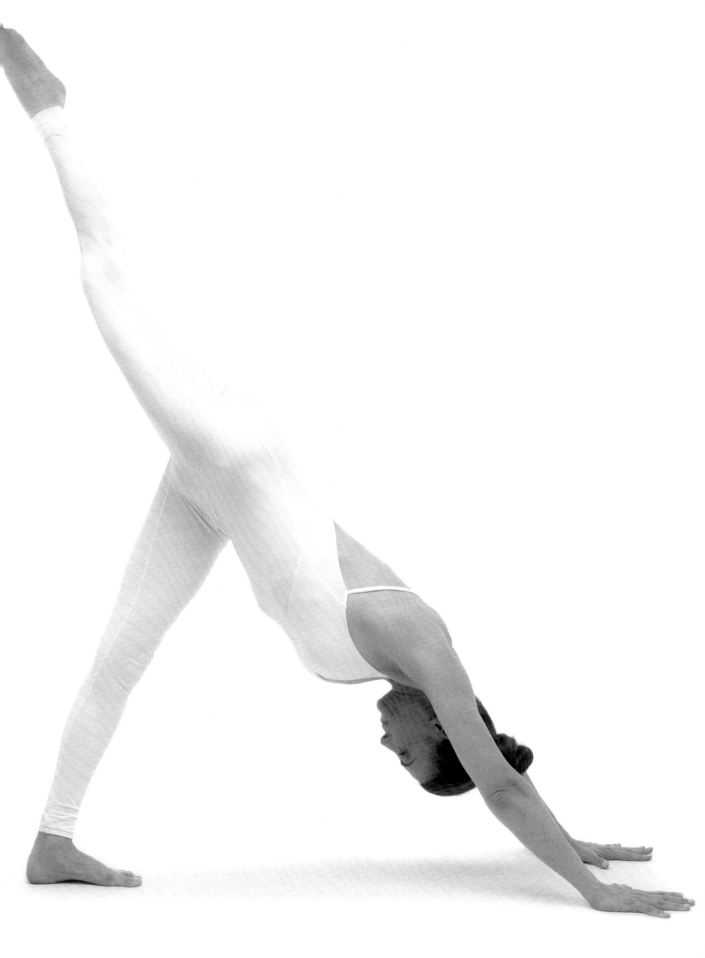

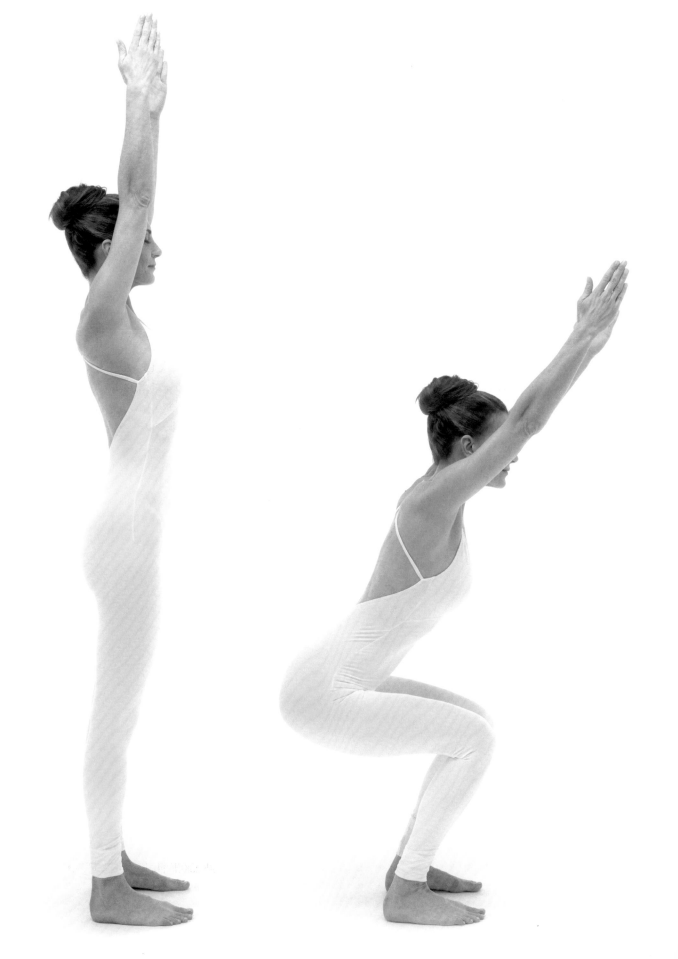

○ CHAIR POSE

Another great exercise to practice daily is Chair Pose. Yogi Bhajan said he practiced this posture every day for three minutes. He raved about this simple posture, and we do as well.

1 Stand up tall, with your legs shoulder width apart. Stretch your arms straight up to the sky, with your palms facing each other.

2 Bend your knees, lower your torso by hinging slightly from your waist, and bring your thighs as parallel to the ground as possible. Draw your shoulder blades down your back and your tailbone down toward the floor.

Make sure your knees do not extend beyond your toes. Keep drawing the glutes back as if you are sitting on a little stool behind you.

3 Breathe deeply and hold the position for as long as you can without straining.

4 To finish, inhale as you come up and straighten your legs. Exhale and stand up tall while breathing deeply and integrating the softness of the breath with the physicality of the exercise. Feel the lightness in your body with the light and illumination of your soul shining around you. Silently say, "I am Light."

MODIFICATION This exercise can be done with a wall behind your back for support. If you are using a wall, press your shoulder blades and spine into the wall as you lower your torso.

○ GODDESS POSE

Goddess Pose is an absolutely incredible exercise for toning the legs and glutes. It also stretches the hips and groins while increasing circulation throughout the body. This pose is excellent for empowering ourselves and feeling the essence of our graceful strength.

If you practice this posture every day for a few weeks, you will see a new tone and feel a newfound strength in your physical body.

1 Stand up tall with your feet three feet apart. Bend your elbows to shoulder height and bring your elbows out to the sides, like the arms of a cactus. Turn the palms to face out in front of you with the fingers spread wide. Turn the toes out forty-five degrees toward the corners of the room and draw your heels closer together.

2 Squat down as far as you can without dropping your hips lower than your knees. Bend your knees out over your toes. Drop your shoulders and draw your neck back. Open your heart and press your chest forward while keeping your chin parallel to the floor.

3 Taking long, slow breaths into your abdomen, hold the posture for as long as you can without straining. Embrace your soft beauty in the midst of the challenging posture. Use your breath to sustain your strength. Feel your grace and allow it to uplift your spirits.

4 When you are ready, inhale and slowly straighten your legs to bring yourself back to an upright position.

5 Exhale and bring your feet together. Relax in a standing position for a few breaths to integrate the physical pose you've just done with your energy. Relax your shoulders while pressing your feet into the earth, elongating your body to the top of your head.

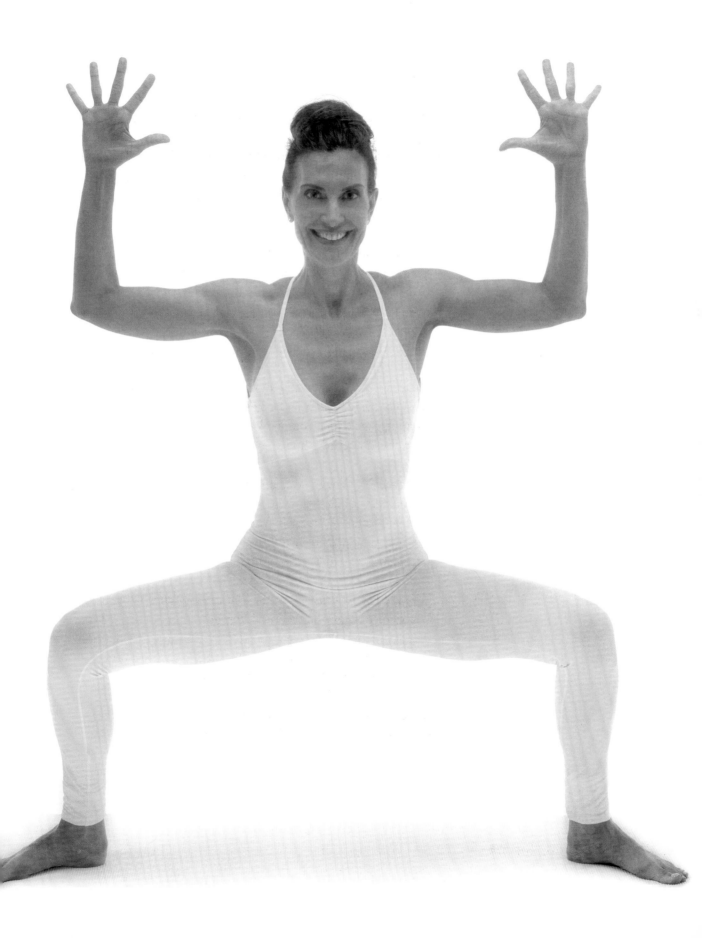

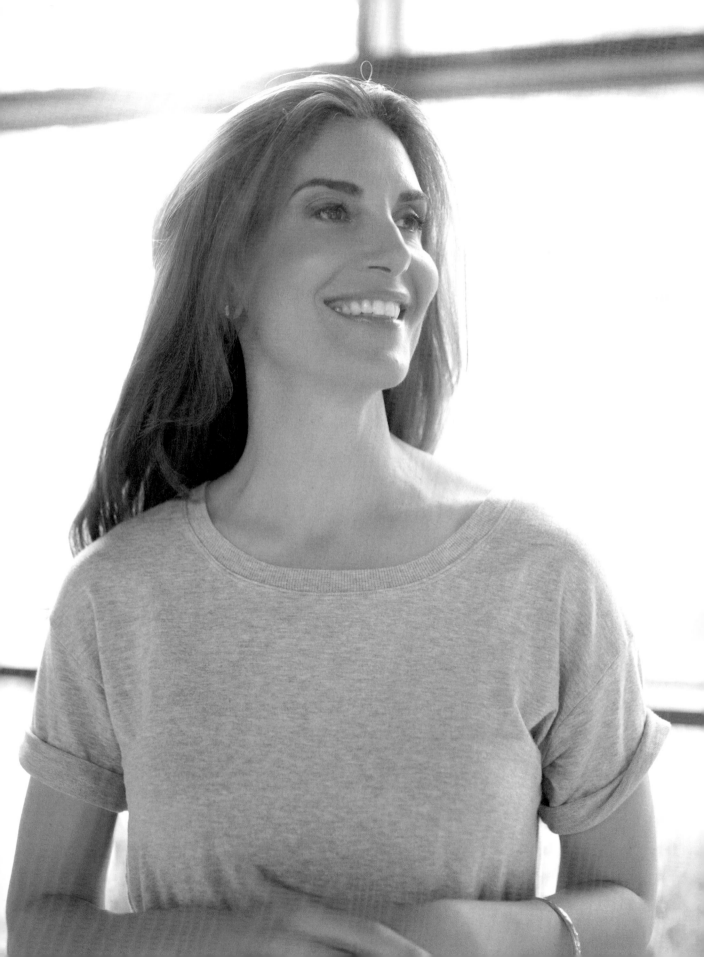

11 KUNDALINI SECRETS FOR HEALTH, BEAUTY, AND VITALITY

For attractive lips, speak words of kindness. For lovely eyes, seek out the good in people. For a slim figure, share your food with the hungry. For beautiful hair, let a child run his fingers through it once a day. For poise, walk with the knowledge you'll never walk alone.
AUDREY HEPBURN

THE MOST ATTRACTIVE PART OF you is your radiance. When our cells are vibrating in alignment with grace and our aura is free of the dullness and density of old mental constructs, we exude a beauty that comes from the magnificence of our soul. We can apply makeup, put on nice clothes, and get our hair styled, which are fun things to do. But if we do not have the inner-to-outer shine, all the fashion in the world will not make us attractive. People who project radiance will be captivating no matter what clothes they are wearing. Although this topic could form the basis of a whole

309

separate book, we chose some of our favorites ways to optimize your attractive nature to share with you here.

COLD SHOWER

Taking cold showers is one of the best things we can do for our health, longevity, and radiance. The cold water brings a burst of circulation to the millions of capillaries in the massive area of the skin, clearing away toxins, bringing oxygen to your body, and resulting in a glowing radiance. The increased circulation helps deep inside the body as well, flushing the inner organs and rejuvenating our blood supply directly from our core.

In kundalini yoga we recommend that you shower before your yoga session. Also, it is recommended that women who are menstruating or pregnant use lukewarm rather than cold water.

Before you take a cold shower, first massage your entire body with pure almond oil, using a circular motion. Turn the water to cold, step into the shower, and let the water hit your feet first, then your legs, and finally your torso. Rub your skin everywhere the water hits. Stay in long enough for your body to adjust to the cold. When you step out of the shower, rub yourself all over with a towel to exfoliate the dead cells from the surface of your skin. Then wrap yourself in warm clothes. You may notice that the cold shower actually warms your body. It really is an awesome feeling, and it gives skin and hair a bewildering glow.

APPLE CIDER BATH

An apple cider bath will release and pull toxins out of your body and your energy field. Draw a hot bath and add two cups of organic apple cider to the water. Get into the bath and state the following affirmation out loud for two minutes: "I am releasing the energy I have absorbed from others, and I am reclaiming my positive energy!" Sit in this bath for at least three minutes. When you're ready, rinse off in a warm shower while imagining all the toxins going down the drain. Then finish by rinsing yourself with cold water, which tightens the pores and seals your energy with your own brightness.

RELAXATION TO CLEAR TOXINS

One of the most effective ways to achieve radiant beauty is to clear metabolic wastes from inside the body on an everyday basis before they can dull our radiance and increase our aging. Eleven minutes of Deep Relaxation is said to release as many toxins from our system as an hour of sleep. Deep Relaxation after a yoga set also clears the subconscious more deeply than even eight hours of sleep can. So do not skip the opportunity to relax on your back for a few minutes, not only after doing a kundalini yoga exercise but anytime you are able. Simply lie down, close your eyes, turn your palms upward, and breathe deeply into your abdomen. For more about Deep Relaxation, please see chapter 6.

FOOD

The secret ingredient in my recipes is one simple thing: love.
GIULIO FERRARI

Karena's father moved to America from Italy when he was in his twenties, and he was such a talented cook that restaurants in New York's Little Italy used to call him in to prepare food for their special guests. Yet Giulio never once went to a cooking class. When people asked him how he prepared his most popular dishes, he would explain in his strong Italian accent that it was with a pinch of this and a pinch of that, but the main ingredient was love.

Vibration is the essential ingredient of healthy food. Your food carries prana into your body. We can't overemphasize the importance of putting love into your cooking. If we were to compare the benefits of organic kale prepared by someone angry versus starchy white pasta made by someone who puts all their love into the food, we would say that the white pasta is in many ways more nourishing and the kale is to be avoided. The vibration of love carried in the molecular structure of food becomes integrated into the molecular structure of your body and into your consciousness.

In general, look for foods that carry a high, fresh, living vibration. The prana carried by fruits, nuts, grains, and vegetables that grow on trees and plants high off the ground will infuse you with sun energy and help keep your prana vibrating at its highest frequency potential. Adding the trinity roots, onions, ginger, and garlic, will give you the sustaining power of mother earth and keep your prana fresh, vibrant, and clean.

No matter what you eat, prepare your food with love and bless your food, your water, and yourself with a prayer before eating, so you take only blessed, high-energy substances into your body. It is important to let go of fanaticism with food as well. The worry and shame of eating unhealthy food can be more harmful than the food itself. Embrace yourself and enjoy eating slowly with people you love. Allow yourself the pleasure of sitting down for a meal with quiet or peaceful conversation. Soft music and candles are a lovely way to enhance the experience as well.

HYDRATION

We all know the importance of drinking water, yet we do not always take this practice seriously enough. Did you know that if you feel thirsty, your body has actually reached a state of dehydration? Make a habit of drinking a tall glass of water after brushing your teeth every morning. Then fill a sixty-four-ounce glass container with water and bring it with you for the day. Drink from it throughout the day so that by the end of your day it is empty. This is a simple and extremely important lifestyle change for those of you who put off drinking water. Water speeds up the metabolism, fuels the brain, and helps the body flush out toxins.

WEIGHT LOSS TEA

A great recipe to jump-start a healthier lifestyle is the weight loss tea below. This ancient tea formula was recommended to dissolve fatty tissue from our bodies and clear toxins from our skin and digestive system. It brings effervescence and beautiful tone to the complexion, giving us a youthful glow. The condition of our skin is correlated with the condition of our digestion. It helps our liver as well. Please note that the recipe calls for black salt, a sea salt from the South Indian Sea revered for centuries as a tonic. It contains a naturally occurring sulphur, giving it a strong taste and smell, so do not use too much.

> ½ cup fresh or dried mint leaves
> 1 cup cumin seeds
> 1 ounce fresh, frozen, or bottled tamarind paste
> ½ teaspoon black salt
> 8 lemons, cut into quarters
> 1 tablespoon whole black peppercorns
> 5 quarts filtered or spring water

Place the ingredients a large pot and let the mixture boil gently for at least fifteen minutes. Then strain and serve hot or cold. Drink a cup early in the morning on an empty stomach and two to three additional cups during the day to cleanse your body of toxins. You may store it refrigerated in a metal, ceramic, or glass container for up to one week. It can be reheated.

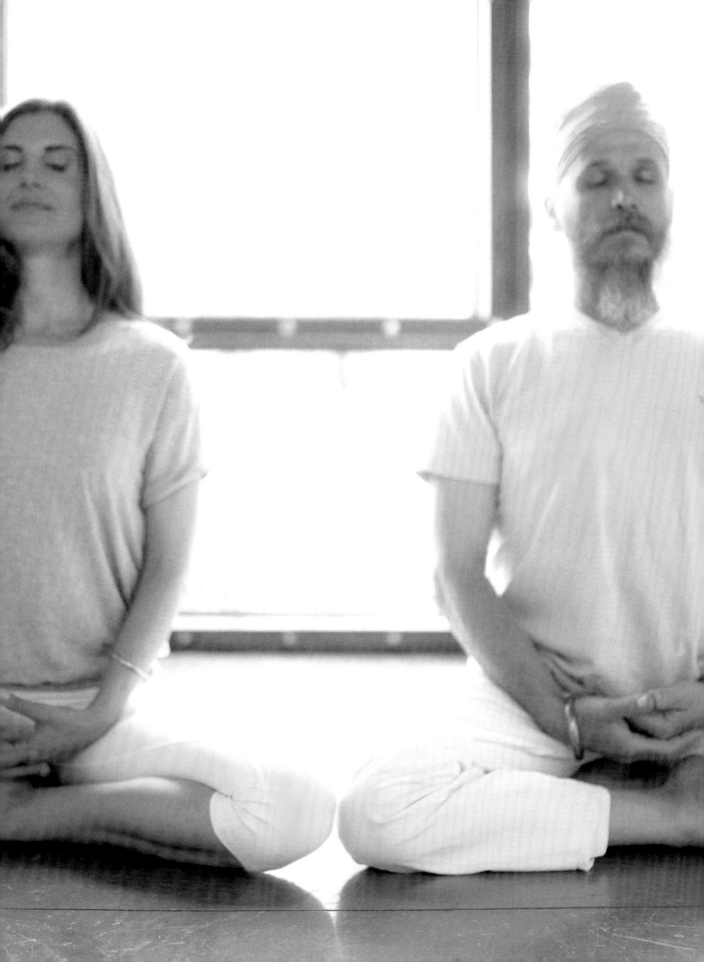

12 INTEGRATING PERSONAL EVOLUTION INTO OUR LIVES

Vibrate the cosmos, and the cosmos shall clear the path.
YOGI BHAJAN

SERVING IN ORDER TO UPLIFT others creates a powerful energy that courses through our being. When we bring love into the world, we ourselves receive as well. In the kundalini tradition, giving selflessly in service to the upliftment of others is called *Seva*. Seva is giving without regard for reward and without need for recognition. The miracle this creates in our psyche cannot be overstated.

Seva is how we take all the benefits of the kundalini yoga practice and put them into action. We roll up our sleeves and get involved with our family, our community, or planet earth. We connect and take action that is inspired by our soul.

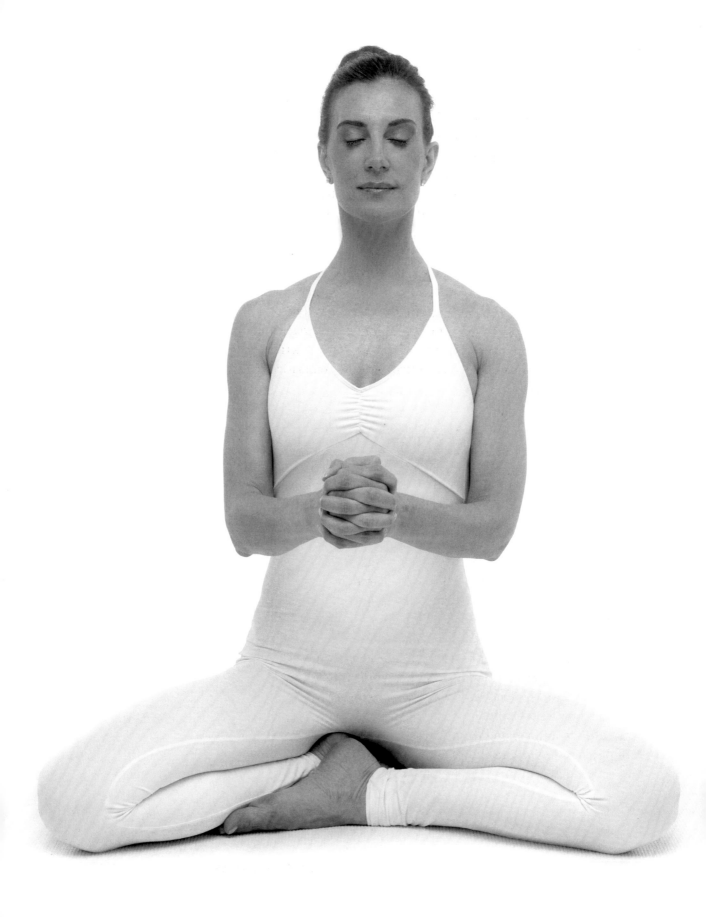

Our souls thrive on giving love. Ever notice how great you feel after helping another? Ever notice the sadness that can envelop you when you are holding back from expressing your love because you are afraid it will not be returned? If we give up on love because others have been hateful, we hurt ourselves. The false beliefs harm us and create constriction rather than expansion. Holding back our love hurts us more than taking a chance and sharing love with others.

We mistakenly believe that we live in a world of scarcity, when in fact our world is full of abundance. There is enough for everyone. There is beauty in seeing the light in others while remembering that we are all part of the same network on earth. When we see the beauty in another, we can recognize that same beauty within ourselves. By shining with authenticity and living into that truth, we give others permission to shine as well. Kundalini practice is your self-care that will strengthen and clarify healthy boundaries for when they are needed.

○ BECOME A CHANNEL TO UPLIFT OTHERS

This is one of our favorite meditations because it actually repairs the aura. There is no other way to become whole except by being a channel that uplifts others.

1 Sit up straight and feel the flow of your breath. Tune in to the flow of breath through your nose and reaching deep into your abdomen. Close your eyes and focus internally on the third eye point.

2 Fold your hands in front of your solar plexus, with the bases of your palms touching and fingers interlaced. Place your elbows alongside your body so that they touch your ribs.

3 Continue taking long, slow, deep, conscious breaths. Inhale as slowly as you can, feeling that God is coming into you

through the breath. Feel the guidance of God. Hold the breath in, then exhale as slowly as you can. Hold the breath out.

4 Mentally expand your awareness of your radiance. See yourself dividing into thirty trillion cells, like sparks dancing from you to the universe. Tell them: "Touch the heart of the one who needs God's help." Allow the energy of the divine to take over. Ask for the highest vibration to come. Surrender and let source be the doer. Continue for three to eleven minutes.

When we activate the Love Frequency Phenomenon, we find our passion for life returns. We are filled with energy when we recognize our calling is to love. The greatest need we have at this time is to unlock the heart and allow love to shine forth. We can become tired and cranky when we see life as a struggle. However, there is nothing to strive for when love is present. Life unfolds with wonder and mystery, even in the greatest of challenges. By vibrating at a frequency of love, you can cultivate greater miracles than you can even imagine. It is the energetic frequency that opens up your God-given potentials for creativity, health, attraction, and inner peace.

We pray that with the guidance from this book you will dust off your diamond and sparkle on with love—thus giving God the greatest compliment possible. Pure light can never be extinguished. Fire can burn out, but pure light only expands. Only density can prevent expansion. Light can never be stopped! Everything but light and love is simply an illusion. You are unstoppable. Receive it. Believe it. Own it. Trust it.

May you feel the love of the divine in every cell of your body.
May this book embrace you in a nurturing light that penetrates deeply into your soul.
May the words create a tangible cloak of peace that envelops and nurtures you, comforts you when you feel alone, and may you always know how very loved you are.
May the divine bless us all as we take this journey together.

With all the love in our hearts,
Karena and Dharm

LISTS OF EXERCISES AND MANTRAS

EXERCISES IN ORDER OF APPEARANCE

ALPHABETICAL LIST OF EXERCISES

LIST OF MANTRAS IN ORDER OF APPEARANCE

RESOURCES FOR FURTHER STUDY

Yogi Bhajan, *The Aquarian Teacher: KRI International Kundalini Yoga Teacher Training Level One*

> (Santa Cruz, NM: Kundalini Research Institute, 2003)
>
> Golden Light Breath, (Yogic Breath), 92
>
> Camel Pose, 312
>
> Guru Pranam, 314
>
> Front Platform, 18
>
> Breath of Fire, 95; 328
>
> Segmented Breath, 97
>
> Miracle Mantra, 84
>
> Mantra for Ecstasy of Consciousness, Wahe Guru, 87
>
> Mul Mantra, 85
>
> Ek Ong Kar Sat Gur Prasad, 84
>
> Cat-Cow, 317
>
> Bow Pose, 317
>
> Frog Pose, 315
>
> Baby Pose, 311
>
> Aura Charger, 314
>
> Stretch Pose, 321
>
> Ad Guray Nameh, 82
>
> Meditation for Healing Self and Others, Ra Ma Da Sa, 86
>
> Long, Deep Breathing (Yogic Breath), 92
>
> Cold Showers, 248–249

Yogi Bhajan, *The Aquarian Teacher: Level One Instructor Manual*

> (Santa Cruz, NM: Kundalini Research Institute, 2003)
>
> Pituitary Gland Series for Intuition, 47

Yogi Bhajan, *Kundalini Yoga/ Sadhana Guidelines*

> (Pomona, CA: Kundalini Research Institute, 1974)
>
> Sat Nam, 38
>
> Long Sat Nam, Seven Wave Sat Nam Meditation, 93
>
> Adi Mantra, 37
>
> Root Lock, Mul Bhand, 41
>
> Diaphragm Lock, Uddiyana Bhand, 41
>
> Neck Lock, Jalandhara Bhand, 41
>
> Great Lock, Maha Bhand, 41
>
> Sat Kriya, 44
>
> Gyan Mudra, 34
>
> Prayer Pose, 35
>
> Venus Lock, 35
>
> Spinal Energy Activation, Basic Spinal Energy Series, 45
>
> Strengthening the Aura to Attract, Strengthening the Aura, 59
>
> Kirtan Kriya, 95–96

Yogi Bhajan, *Kundalini Yoga for Youth and Joy*

> (Eugene, OR: 3HO Transcripts, 1983)
>
> Lion Claw Exercise to Reset Your Magnetic Field, 13

Yogi Bhajan, *Praana, Praanee, Praanayam: Exploring the Breath Technology of Kundalini Yoga as Taught by Yogi Bhajan*

> (Santa Cruz, NM: Kundalini Research Institute, 2006)
>
> Breath for Intuition, 162–163

Harijot Kaur Khalsa, *Physical Wisdom*

> (Española, NM: Kundalini Research Institute, 1994)
>
> Heart Centering Meditation, 35

Guru Nanak, Japji Sahib

> (14th Century, transliterated by the authors)
>
> Mul Mantra

Exercises from personal experience, traditional yogic practices, conceived by the authors, or without documented sources:

> Expand Your Electromagnetic Frequency
>
> Vocalization in Camel Pose
>
> Crow Pose
>
> Pelvic Lifts
>
> Alternate Nostril Breathing
>
> Square Breath
>
> Thoracic Nerve Stimulation
>
> Sacral Nerve Activation
>
> Whistling Breath for Vagas Nerve
>
> Vitality Stretch
>
> Power Archer
>
> The Divine Grind
>
> Miracle Breath
>
> Ma
>
> Connect with the Sound of the Soul
>
> Deep Relaxation
>
> Advanced Cat-Cow with Knee Bend
>
> Exercise for Auric Sensitivity
>
> Stretching Exercise

Yoga for the Spine and Immune System

Patience Pays Affirmation

The Advance Gratitude Technique

Meditation for Releasing Shame

Elixir for Calm

Kundalini Yoga to Dissolve the Barriers of Fear

Fertility Visualization

Fertility Dance

Triangle with Reverse Leg Lifts

Chair Pose

Goddess Pose

Relaxation to Clear Toxins

Meditation for Guruprasad

(*Aquarian Times Magazine*, Nov/Dec 2007)

Meditation for Guru Prasad

Meditation Course

Yogi Bhajan Library of Teachings, accessed on July 17, 2016. http://www.libraryofteachings.com/lecture.xqy?q=date:1976-10-20&id=6cc61d15-2d14-cb2b-6370-f0fac9380335&title=Meditation-Course

Mindful Centering, Nadi Sodhni

KWTC - Kundalini Yoga

Yogi Bhajan Library of Teachings, accessed July 17, 2016. http://libraryofteachings.com/lecture.xqy?q=date:1984-07-05&id=1dc2d184-95b3-4359-f95c-3d21c95fb4bc&title=KWTC---Kundalini-Yoga

Kriya for Going with the Flow

Kundalini Yoga

The Yogi Bhajan Library of Teachings, accessed July 17, 2016. http://www.libraryofteachings.com/lecture.xqy?q=date:1984-10-31&id=74bf2059-2107-5b28-e3aa-9073e53ffc5f&title=Kundalini-Yoga

Detoxing for Radiance

Advanced Class

The Yogi Bhajan Library of Teachings, accessed July 17, 2016. http://www.libraryofteachings.com/lecture.xqy?q=date:1974-05-27&id=a87aab01-6abc-2227-f422-1ee6e3b5920e&title=Advanced-Class

Meditation for Guidance, Waho Guru

Longevity Kriya

Kundalini Research Institute, accessed July 17, 2016. http://www.kundalinirising.org/KRIResource/Kriyas/LongevityKriya.pdf

Longevity Kriya

Meditation for Release of Cold Depression

(From lecture by Yogi Bhajan dated October 17, 2000. Printed in *Aquarian Times Magazine*, Winter 2001)

Cold Depression Meditation

Meditation for Becoming a Channel to Uplift Others in the Aquarian Age

Khalsa Coucil - SSS Address, Kundalini Research Institute, accessed August 26, 2016. http://www.libraryofteachings.com/lecture.xqy?q=date:1998-04-10&id=13977c84-009c-3364-5328-88470219cc42&title=Khalsa-Council---SSS-Address---Day-3---Contains-Meditation

Become a Channel to Uplift Others

Children

Yogi Bhajan Library of Teachings, accessed on August 26, 2016. http://www.libraryofteachings.com/lecture.xqy?q=date:1989-02-03&id=1b236d62-f15b-8b6b-9f8a-d4d3d47cdeae&title=Children

Flow and Glow

Yogi Bhajan, *I Am a Woman: Creative, Sacred & Invincible—Essential Kriyas For Women In The Aquarian Age*

(Santa Cruz, NM: Kundalini Research Institute, 2009)

Breathing to Clear Emotions from the Past

Meditation Course

The Yogi Bhajan Library of Teachings, accessed on August 26, 2016. http://www.libraryofteachings.com/lecture.xqy?q=date:1989-12-08&id=4acc4c92-ad21-9593-ea96-f35af3413692&title=Meditation-Course---Day-One

Activating Healing

Kundalini Yoga for the Skin

Kundalini Research Institute, accessed July 17, 2016. http://www.libraryofteachings.com/lecture.xqy?q=date:1986-02-26&id=be3c2c57-3460-7073-2832-9a9adb822b52&title=Kundalini-Yoga---For-the-Skin

Kriya for Radiant Skin

AUTHORS' NOTE

IN THIS BOOK, WE HAVE carefully chosen techniques that we have found to be most powerful in our own practices and as inspired from the classes, writing, and personal instruction of Yogi Bhajan. Our intention is to honor the accuracy of how these practices were originally explained by Yogi Bhajan and, at the same time, include helpful and instructive details for the methods and insights that we have found beneficial in getting the most from these powerful techniques. These details are based on our notes, experience with Yogi Bhajan, and decades of working with these techniques. In order to keep this clear to our readers, the full sequences known as "sets" are per Yogi Bhajan, while many of the nuanced instructions, as well as the titles, were written and nicknamed by the authors.

We have also made a point of adding "tuning in with mindful centering," deep breathing, the Adi Mantra, use of an energy locks, and Deep Relaxation, whether or not they were part of the original classes. Where we have added suggestions and techniques based on our own experience or other sources will be indicated with the terms "invite," "suggest," or "visualize." We have suggested modifications for many of the more challenging exercises that offer the benefits of the technique in a less strenuous position, even though modifications were generally not part of Yogi Bhajan's original classes. By the way, the best modification, if you simply can't do a particular exercise in this book, is simply to lie down on your back and visualize your body in the exercise. This will stimulate many portions of the brain and nervous system, and generate many of the positive effects that actually performing an exercise does. In all cases, the original sources, where available, are listed in the resources section, so you can look them up for further study.

ACKNOWLEDGMENTS

WE WOULD LIKE TO THANK so many people for their unwavering support, love, nurturing, devotion, and individual sparks of God. We are so grateful for the beauty that happens when hearts come together in a vibration that shares healing with the world. This book is so much bigger than us; it has been a task of the heart, and it would not have been possible without the support of so many.

Thank you to the entire team at Sounds True for believing in this project, and for your guidance and wisdom in planning and executing this creation, especially Jennifer Brown, Tami Simon, Jade Lascelles, Amy Rost, Diana Rico, Rachael Murray, Brooks Freehill, Jen Murphy, Beth Skelley, Anastasia Pellouchoud, Karen Polaski, Matt Howe, and Cynthia Moore.

To Yogi Bhajan for delivering these teachings and his loving presence in our lives. Thank you to KRI for holding the teachings of kundalini yoga with such integrity, especially Nirvair Singh and Siri Neel Kaur.

To our families for their love and support: Beryl, Giulio, Robert, Karen, Otello, and Stephanie Ferrari; Charles, Gabriella, and Christian Virginia; Gurukirn Kaur, Hari Rai, and Sahib Simran Khalsa; Osa Skotting Maclane, and Irving Segal, William and Karen Segal.

To the network of those who have held us while touching our souls, some since childhood: Swami Janakanda, Mr. Drake, Ms. Gay and Ms. Langsdorf, Frances Foden, Dorothy and Roy James, Sue and Ali Meier, Peter James, Elaine Welchman, Sheila Bates, Carole Hannon, Kathy Dellanno, Michele Nunziato, Nina Grasso, Sandra DelCioppio, Snatam Kaur, Maha Atma Singh, Shakti Parwha Kaur, Debbie Diament, Nirinjan Kaur, Jeanne Glynn, William Kelly, and Bruce Springsteen.

We would also thank the beautiful angels who have guided us to serve everyone who reads this book so it can be a gift of light, uplifting, and grace. We thank all of you who are holding this book and trusting the blessings of this sacred design. May the Divine bless us all as we hold hands and walk together… forever.

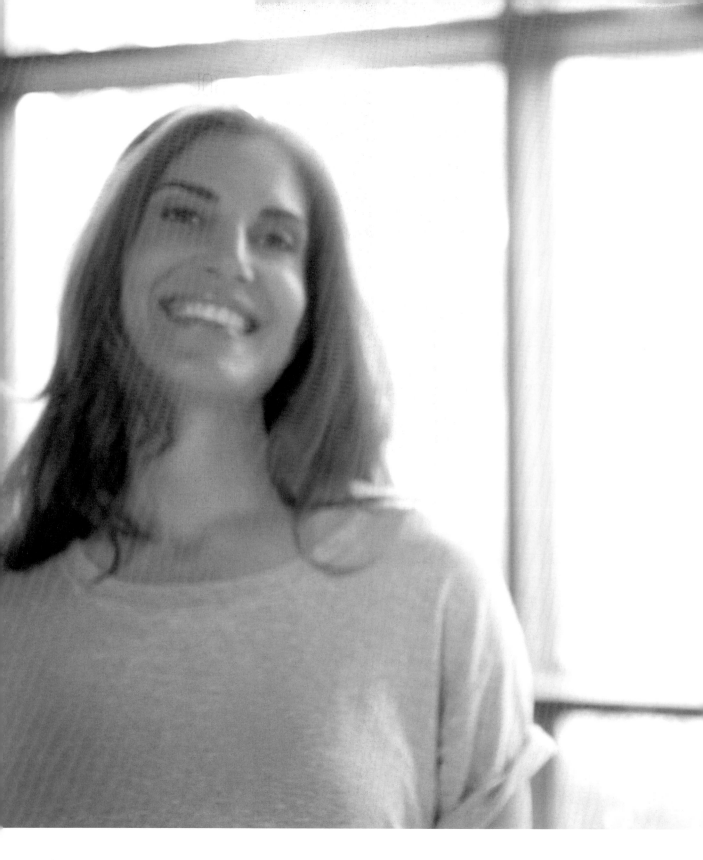

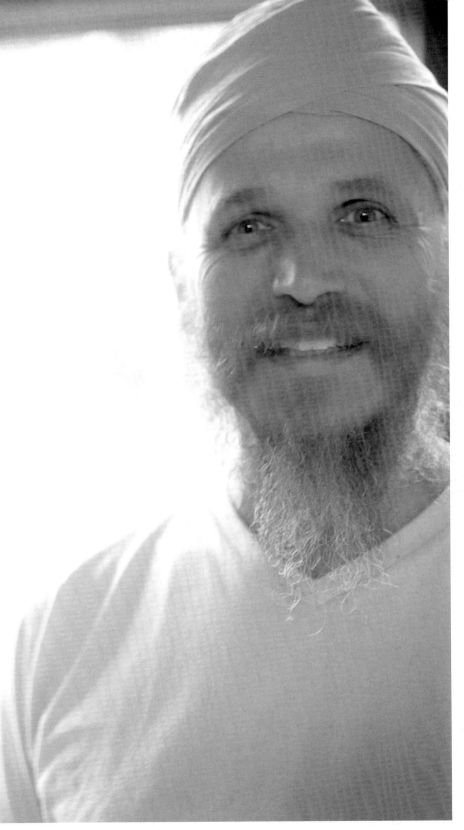

ABOUT THE AUTHORS

KARENA VIRGINIA is a deeply spiritual life coach, inspirational speaker, healer, yoga teacher, and TV personality. A graduate of Ithaca College and former actor and model, Karena found through experience that mindfulness and love is the key to life fulfillment. She has been teaching and speaking throughout the United States and Europe explaining the law of attraction and kundalini yoga in a very basic, clear, and scientific way. She is known for her transformational and accessible messages which bring powerful and mystical practices to the mainstream. Karena believes we are living in a profound time of miracles and that living through the heart with grace, peace, truth, flow, and light while uplifting others is the surest path to attracting the life of our dreams. Karena's other work includes the highly acclaimed DVD *The Power of Kundalini Yoga* and the app *Relax and Attract with Karena*. Karena has been featured on Veria Living and Bravo TV along with various wellness publications around the world. She is a member of Oprah Winfrey's Belief team, and her passion is to bring her message of simple everyday healing to people around the globe. Karena can currently be found on daytime television sharing lifestyle and wellness tips with a modern flair. Raised by European parents, she resides in the suburbs of New York City with her husband and two children. For more information about Karena, visit her website: karenavirginia.com.

DHARM KHALSA is on the board of trustees of the Siri Singh Sahib Corporation—the non-profit organization that oversees kundalini yoga in the United States after the passing of Yogi Bhajan in 2004—as well as 3HO Foundation and Unto Infinity. He has been teaching kundalini yoga since 1980 and was a close student and staff member of Yogi Bhajan. He is a second generation yoga teacher, having first learned Iyengar style yoga from his mother, Osa Skotting Maclane. He was born as Andrew Segal in Copenhagen, Denmark, to his visionary artist mother and leading mathematics professor father, Irving Segal. He grew up in Massachusetts and is a graduate of the University of Rochester with a BA in psychology. He became sevadar to Yogi Bhajan in 1982, adopting the spiritual name Dharm Khalsa, and serving and learning directly from Yogi Bhajan in Los Angeles for many years. He leads early morning meditations, has recorded four albums of mantra music, is a minister of the Sikh faith, and travels and teaches workshops primarily in the United States and Europe. He believes that when we live in our truth from the heart there is an awareness of love that flows like a current through all things. Recognizing that current of love provides the framework for a life of fulfillment, joy, and meaning. Dharm currently resides in the kundalini ashram community of Española, New Mexico, with his wife and two daughters. For more information about Dharm, his website is dharmji.com.

ABOUT SOUNDS TRUE

SOUNDS TRUE IS A MULTIMEDIA publisher whose mission is to inspire and support personal transformation and spiritual awakening. Founded in 1985 and located in Boulder, Colorado, we work with many of the leading spiritual teachers, thinkers, healers, and visionary artists of our time. We strive with every title to preserve the essential "living wisdom" of the author or artist. It is our goal to create products that not only provide information to a reader or listener, but that also embody the quality of a wisdom transmission.

For those seeking genuine transformation, Sounds True is your trusted partner. At SoundsTrue.com you will find a wealth of free resources to support your journey, including exclusive weekly audio interviews, free downloads, interactive learning tools, and other special savings on all our titles.

To learn more, please visit SoundsTrue.com/freegifts or call us toll-free at 800.333.9185.

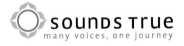